First Aid for Beginners

Learn How to Act in an Emergency Situation, and Provide First Aid to the Injured Until Help Arrives

Author: Pamela C. Walker

© Copyright 2020 - All rights reserved.

The content contained within this book may not be reproduced, duplicated or transmitted without direct written permission from the author or the publisher.

Under no circumstances will any blame or legal responsibility be held against the publisher, or author, for any damages, reparation, or monetary loss due to the information contained within this book, either directly or indirectly.

Legal Notice:

This book is copyright protected. It is only for personal use. You cannot amend, distribute, sell, use, quote or paraphrase any part, or the content within this book, without the consent of the author or publisher.

Disclaimer Notice:

Please note the information contained within this document is for educational and entertainment purposes only. All effort has been executed to present accurate, up to date, reliable, complete information. No warranties of any kind are declared or implied. Readers acknowledge that the author is not engaging in the rendering of legal, financial, medical or professional advice. The content within this book has been derived from various sources. Please consult a licensed professional before attempting any techniques outlined in this book.

By reading this document, the reader agrees that under no circumstances is the author responsible for any losses, direct or indirect, that are incurred as a result of the use of information contained within this document, including, but not limited to, errors, omissions, or inaccuracies.

Free Gift

This book includes a bonus booklet. This giveaway may be for a limited time only. All information on how you can secure your gift right now can be found at the end of this book.

Table of Content

BOOK DESCRIPTION 3
INTRODUCTION 4
GLOSSARY 6
CHAPTER 1 UNDERSTANDING THE
BASICS OF FIRST AID 11
    Understanding First Aid Basics (ABCs of First Aid) 11
    First Aid Steps (The 3Cs) 12
        First C – Check 13
        Second C – Call 13
        Third C – Care 13
    Qualities of a Good First Aider 14
    Roles and Responsibilities of a First Aider 15
    First Aid Myths and Common Mistakes 17
CHAPTER 2 FIRST AID KIT ESSENTIALS 23
    A Basic First Aid Kit 23
    Types of First Aid Kits 27
        Home First Aid Kits 27
        Travel First Aid Kits 28
        Office First Aid Kits 31
        Camping First Aid Kits 32
        Disaster First Aid Kits 34
CHAPTER 3 RECOGNIZING EMERGENCIES 38

What Counts as a Medical Emergency? 38
    Listen for Any Unusual Sounds *39*
    Look for any Unusual Sights *40*
    Sense any Unusual Smell *40*
    Notice any Unusual Behavioral Change *41*
Warning Signs of a Medical Emergency 42
    Is it An Urgent Medical Emergency? *44*

CHAPTER 4 PROVIDING FIRST AID AROUND INFECTIOUS DISEASES 47

Precautionary Gear Essentials 47
    Gloves *48*
    CPR Adjunct *48*
The Risks 49
Precautions to Take Around the Patient 50
Disinfection of Contaminated Areas 51
Precautions for Dealing with Body Fluids Spillages 53

CHAPTER 5 FIRST AID TECHNIQUES 101 55

Using a Defibrillator (AED) 55
Resuscitation 57
    Babies *57*
    Children and Adults *59*
CPR 60
    Performing CPR: The How-To *61*
Dressing a Wound 63
Bandaging a Wound 67
    Roller Bandages *68*
    Triangular Bandages *68*
    Tubular Bandages *69*

Steps to Bandaging 69

CHAPTER 6 14 BASIC FIRST-AID PROCEDURES EVERYONE SHOULD KNOW 73

Cardiac Arrest 73

Choking 74

Sprains 76

Frostbite 77

Nosebleed 78

Allergic Reactions 79

Bee Sting 81

Heatstroke 82

Cuts and Scrapes 83

Bleeding 83

Fracture 84

Blisters 85

Burns 86

Jellyfish Stings 87

CHAPTER 7 MEDICAL CONDITIONS REQUIRING IMMEDIATE HELP 89

Heart Attack 89

What to Do? 90

Stroke 91

What to Do? 92

Angina 93

What to Do? 94

Drowning 95

What to Do? 95

v

Dislocation of Bones 96
    What to Do? *97*
Seizures 98
    What to Do? *99*
Childbirth 100
    What to Do *101*

FINAL THOUGHTS 103
DOWNLOAD YOUR FREE GIFT BELOW: 105
CHECK OUT OUR OTHER *AMAZING* TITLES: 107

Legal Matters 108
    Power of Attorneys *108*
    Financial Aspects *110*
    Emergency Guardianship *111*
    Hiring an Attorney *111*
Medical Matters 113
    Costs *114*
Safety and Your Home 115
    Prep Hotspots *116*
    Kitchens *116*
    Know Your Numbers *117*
    Check Your Safety Devices *117*
    Install Locks Wisely *117*
    Light it Up *118*
    Remove Any Weapons *118*
    Store Medication *118*
    Tripping Hazards *118*
Bodyweight Training; Getting Started 125
    Full Body *126*

Legs *128*
Back and Chest *129*
Shoulders and Arms *130*
REFERENCES **132**

These 14 New Habits Will Double Your Income, from Today

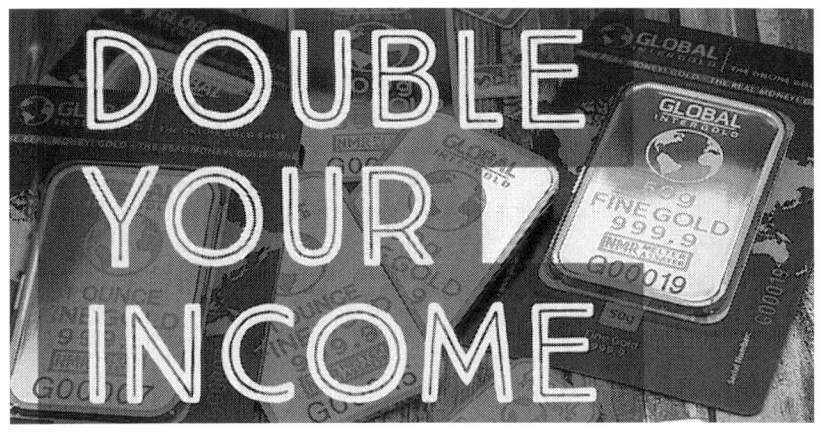

An Easy Cheat Sheet to Adopting 14 Powerful Success Habits:

Stop Procrastinating and Start Earning with Intent Now!

Are Your Bad Habits Keeping You from the Life You Want?

Mine definitely were, but then I dedicated myself to *new habits* – and everything changed!

Most people get stuck in same old routines. We eat the same breakfast, we talk to the same people. Human beings are creatures of habit, and it locks us into negative cycles we don't even know are there. Like me, you've had enough of the same-old, same-old. It's time for change!

This guide gives you the 14 most high impact habits that helped me double my income nearly instantly, when I set out on this journey. I will help you change, and I'll make it stick!

First Aid for Beginners

This FREE Cheat Sheet contains:

- Daily success habits that the most successful people in the world live by

- Common, but little-known habits that will surprise you

- Details on what Stephen Covey, Oprah Winfrey, Elon Musk, Bill Gates and Albert Einstein did that you aren't doing to maximize your earning potential

- Tips on how to overcome habit fatigue

- The reality of adopting difficult, challenging habits and the rewards that result

Scroll below and <u>click the link to claim</u> your cheat sheet!

It's tough to admit that you're doing it wrong. I went through it, and it sucks. After that I was free to change however necessary, to meet my goals. I want you to know that change is waiting for you. This guide is so easy to follow, and if you put it to work in your life – you will double your income.

Adopt these habits, and change your life.

<u>CLICK HERE!!</u>

Book Description

Everyone must know basic first aid. In times, when accidents can happen in seconds, one must learn basic first aid. Lucky for you, in this guide, the readers can find how to deal with some of the most common and everyday incidents like a nosebleed, choking, fainting or cuts and scrapes as well as some major health conditions like a heart attack or seizures. Even though the role of any first aider is to prevent the situation from getting worse, it can be extremely helpful to have someone knowledgeable to handle such situations. Learning about how to use an automated external defibrillator, giving chest compressions or taking precautionary measures around blood and other bodily fluids is equally essential.

So the next time you find someone choking, losing consciousness, having a stroke, drowning, screaming from a bee/jellyfish sting or experiencing cardiac arrest, you don't just stop, stare and wait for someone else to help, but rather, you are a helpful resource yourself and administer basic first aid to the victim.

From preparing your beginner's first aid kit to learning how to bandage a wound, you shall find it all in this brief but informative guide. So be the hero next time someone needs medical assistance!

Introduction

First aid refers to immediate or emergency care provided to someone ill or injured before the victim receives full medical treatment. Usually, it is the first point of contact between the victim and the care provider where the first aider tries to contain the situation using some basic procedures such as trying to stop bleeding, laying the patient down, covering the open wound to prevent bacteria or giving artificial ventilation in cases when the victim isn't breathing. For conditions considered minor, such as a bug bite or nausea, first-aid is all that is required. However, in case of mass casualties or serious conditions where a fatality might be expected, first aid must be given continuously until advanced medical care arrives.

Whichever is the case, the decision to act at the right moment can be the difference between life and death. Did you know, according to a hard-hitting advert campaign, St. John Ambulance revealed that 140,000 people lose their lives in situations where basic first aid could have saved them? (Boseley, 2012). It is the same amount of people dying from cancer each year which happens to be the most common worldwide disease. Shocking, no? Imagine having to say goodbye to a loved one just because no one around them knew basic first aid when they needed it the most? Are you willing to live with the guilt that you could have saved a life and didn't?

Therefore, in this time of age where reckless driving, negligence towards children and workplace injuries make the headlines of every newspaper weekly, it is your job to play the responsible party and prevent any injuries from turning into fatalities. The best part, it isn't as complicated as you think!

In this guide, we are going to be covering some of the very basic first-aid techniques, procedures and precautionary tips to prepare you for any unforeseen circumstances.

It will cover topics such as how you can identify between medical and non-medical emergency, how to handle both, how to take precautions around blood, bodily fluids and how to clean contaminated spaces using the supplies in your first aid kit, what procedures you must be aware of and prepared to do, etc.

The goal is to teach you how to transform from a bystander to a first responder. With the knowledge and techniques, you will always have the upper hand when situations go out of control and hopefully save lives.

Let's begin!

This book comes with a FREE Bonus chapter section as a gift. You can download them for free. The free content can be found at the bottom of this book.

Glossary

ABCD of CPR – A is for airway, B is for breathing, C is for circulation, and D is for defibrillation.

Abrasion – Any skin that has been scraped off.

Amputation – Any body part such as the arm or leg that has been separated from the body completely.

Anaphylactic shock – A type of shock in which an individual has an allergic or hypersensitive reaction to medication, food, bites or insect stings.

Avulsion – Tissue that has been torn from the body.

Burn – An injury caused by fire, radiation, heat, chemical agents or electricity. It is measured by the severity and burning of the layers of the skin.

Chest Compressions – It is an act of building pressure on the chest by repeatedly pushing onto the chest during CPR. Chest compressions improve the flow of blood to the heart and the blood vessels.

Contact poisoning – Poisoning that happens when an individual's skin comes in contact with a poisonous substance or chemical.

Convulsion – Convulsion is a type of seizure in which one suffers from involuntary muscle contractions.

CPR – The act of supplying the heart and surrounding blood vessels with enough blood and oxygen to keep it beating. It is an artificial way to keep the heart pumping blood during a cardiac arrest.

Defibrillator – A device that uses electrical shocks to reinstate an individual's normal heartbeat.

Dislocation - A dislocation occurs when one end of the bone is displaced from its original position. Since all bones are secured by joints on each end, when a dislocation occurs, one part of the bone moves out of the joint.

Direct pressure – A technique used to stop bleeding from an open wound.

Dressing – A piece of soft fabric used to cover an injury, wound or body part. It is made from a sterile material and comes in a range of sizes to cater to both big and small wounds.

Ear injuries – Ear injuries happen when there is either perforation or rupture of the eardrum.

Fainting – Fainting is a natural body reaction when the brain lacks blood. As a response, the body drops down to the floor to allow better circulation of the blood to the brain. It is usually a temporary state but can also be a symptom of epilepsy.

Fracture – A fracture means there has been a crack in the bone.

Frostbite – Frostbite is a condition in which one's tissue fluid freeze. It is mostly accompanied by skin tissue damage.

Full-thickness – Full-thickness refers to a third-degree burn which is the most severe kind of burn. It leaves the skin charred, black, or even red. It is the burning of all seven layers of the skin that protects the organs and even cause damage to the underlying tissue.

Head injuries – A head injury refers to any blow or wound on the head or skull.

Heart attack – A heart attack is an immediate incidence of coronary thrombosis which results in the death of heart muscle or a part of it and can be fatal.

Heat cramps – Heat cramps are a result of excessive exposure to heat. They can lead to dehydration as the body loses water and salt via sweat.

Heatstroke – A heatstroke occurs when an individual is exposed to high temperatures for long durations. It can sometimes be fatal as well as it damages the heart, kidneys, and lungs and causes difficulty in breathing.

Hypothermia – It is a state of the body when the temperature goes down from 35° C (95°F).

Incision – An incision is an injury or cut caused by a sharp object.

Laceration – A laceration is the tearing of tissues by force such as an incision made using a knife or blade.

Partial-thickness – Partial-thickness refers to second-degree burns that leave the skin blistered, moist, pink or red.

Personal Protective Equipment (PPE) – This is an essential first aid equipment worn to prevent exposure to hazards. It includes protective clothing, goggles, gloves, and masks to keep the nose and mouth from inhaling toxic gases or harmful chemicals.

Poisoning – Poisoning occurs when an individual ingests something lethal. If the poison isn't treated immediately, it can enter the bloodstream and cause clotting, thus obstructing the flow of blood to the heart.

Puncture – A puncture is a type of wound that happens when something sharp such as a nail, pin or pointed object bursts a hole in any of the organs or skin.

Recovery position – It is a position used mostly during the administration of first aid that allows the injured person to lie in a comfortable position where his/her airways are open and clear so that in case they feel like vomiting, they won't choke.

Resuscitation – Resuscitation refers to the technique of restoring one's life using CPR.

Seizure – A seizure means that an individual's brain has some uncontrollable or abnormal electrical activity. Sometimes, it is also referred to as a convulsion. Seizures are a sign of an underlying health condition such as epilepsy or allergic reaction.

Slings – Slings are a first aid supply which consists of a series of straps for around the neck region or the thoracic region.

Splints – Splints are devices used to immobilize wounded parts when dislocations, fractures, and other bone-related injuries are suspected or have occurred until help arrives.

First Aid for Beginners

Sprain – A sprain is any injury in the tissues of the joints.

Strains – A strain occurs when a muscle has been overstretched without care and thus torn or inflamed.

Superficial – Superficial refers to first-degree burns that leave the skin looking red, dried out and flaky.

Trauma – A trauma is a state in which one suffers from an emotional or physical injury as a result of some terrible accident or event.

Unconscious – It is a state of mind in which the mind is unable to make sense or respond to its surroundings. Think of it as going completely numb. It usually happens when the brain suffers from a lack of oxygen or blood.

Wound - A wound is an injury in the soft tissues. It can either be open or closed. In a closed wound, blood clots around the injured area and stops the flow of blood. When left unattended, it can swell up and cause severe pain.

X-ray – X-ray is a high-energy radiation technique that uses electromagnetic rays to receive clear images of the organs inside the body. It is used to diagnose diseases such as tumors, cancer or obstruction in blood vessels.

Chapter 1
Understanding the Basics of First Aid

"Heroes represent the best of ourselves, respecting that we are human beings. A hero can be anyone from Gandhi to your classroom teacher, anyone who can show courage when faced with a problem. A hero is someone willing to help others in his or her best capacity."

~Ricky Martin

In the first chapter, we shall be discussing what first aid is all about, how to proceed with administering first aid to someone, the roles, and responsibilities of a first aider, the mistakes first aiders often respond with and the myths revolving around it.

Understanding First Aid Basics (ABCs of First Aid)

The first step before any first aid procedure is assessing the situation and the severity of the problem. Remember, you have to help yourself first. This means that if the incident involves any exposure to harmful toxins, chemicals or gas, you must protect yourself first. In cases other than that, you must critically evaluate the situation and recognize and remember all the details of the scene. If the situation involves any use of a weapon or reckless driving, for instance, looking at the assaulter or the owner of the vehicle can help with the filing of the case later. The goal is to help out the victim in every way possible. In case you feel that the victim is severely injured and requires medical attention instantaneously, then try calling 911 or if you are attending the victim, ask someone nearby to make the call. This will activate the process of emergency response. If you aren't sure how to proceed or how serious the condition of the victim is, a 911 representative can ask you a series of questions and help you out as well. Therefore, the first step involves getting the 911 operator on board.

Once you have an operator online, don't drop the line until help arrives. Hanging up the phone will make it harder for the dispatch emergency unit to find you and may take more time. It is best to be as specific as possible about the details of your whereabouts. Plus, the operator is trained to address such queries which means you have a better chance at providing better care to the victim and with more caution and confidence. He/she will guide you through the process of CPR if the victim isn't breathing, teach you how to use an automatic external defibrillator or guide you through the steps of bandaging the victim, all of which will make a huge difference when done right.

Thirdly, you need to have an emergency first aid kit prepared at all times and with you when traveling. If it is a workplace emergency, there are several protocols you will have to follow before you begin with first aid. It is best to be aware of them and also about what you have in your first-aid kit.

First Aid Steps (The 3Cs)

In medical terms, the steps to any first aid attempt are referred to as the 3 C's. Since medical emergencies can happen to anyone at any time, first aiders are expected to perform these 3 steps and in this specific order as described below. Doing so helps both the victim and the medical emergency unit to administer medical help to the injured promptly.

First C – Check

The first step includes checking and analyzing the situation off the accident or emergency. Is it a busy road, is the traffic coming at high speed, is it at a demolished site? Is there a chance of more demolition? Is it at a factory where chemicals or toxic gases have been released? Or is it at your home where you are the only one with the victim? All of these conditions require different protocols. Such as, in the case of a demolition site where further demolition is expected, the first step is to help the victim get away from the area. If it is an infectious or hazardous area where exposure to toxins and chemicals is a possibility, then you need to think about your safety first and later, try to prevent the patient from inhaling those gases and causing more harm, etc.

Second C – Call

Every emergency needs a quick and responsive first aider. The second most crucial step involves getting 911 on board and any emergency numbers you can recall to get the patient to a nearby facility as soon as possible. When the call has been made, check the status of the victim. Is he/she breathing fine, able to tell their name and blood type or any other significant detail about themselves? In case the patient is unconscious, check for a pulse and start CPR.

Third C – Care

Once the call has been made and the situation analyzed, the first responder must administer primary care which may or may not involve giving CPR, stopping the bleeding or helping the patient lie in a comfortable position and assess any fractures or spinal cord injury.

Qualities of a Good First Aider

Although there are a set of qualifications, training, and certifications that earns one the title of a registered first aider, there are some traits that go beyond the knowledge and skills learned on the job. These qualities are what make a first aider stand out. Take a look at them below and you will understand what we are talking about.

A first aider must:

Have Good Communication Skills

It is most important for any first aider to be as communicative as possible. In many situations, the injured is responsive but in a state of shock. A communicative first aider can help them assess the situation better, reassure them that help is on the way and get as many details out of them as possible, such as their medical history and any key details the doctors may find helpful. This channel of communication can also help the patient feel safer and stay calm and composed. Additionally, it also takes their minds off of the trauma they have been in and makes the situation a lot easier for everyone.

Have the Ability to Respond Under Pressure

A standout first aider must also work his/her best under pressure. Sometimes the situation can be as simple as attending to a cut or bee sting and other times it can be as difficult as giving someone CPR to keep them alive. A first aider must be mentally and physically capable and prepared for all sorts of possibilities and be able to keep their cool under all conditions. The more in control the first aider is, the better his/her administering will be.

Be Positive and Assuring

Understandably, the one who has just met with an accident will be scared and confused about the situation. A first aider must be, at all times, positive and reassure the patient from time to time about how good they are doing and that help is on its way. Someone optimistic and calm under pressure would be ideal. Since there is always the possibility of the situation worsening, the first aider must also remain mentally attentive and keep their emotions from overtaking their judgment.

Have Leadership and Good Initiation Skills

Time is of great essence in any medical emergency. Thus, the first aider must be able to respond quickly at all times and lead from the front. He/she must also be able to trust their judgment, not panic and use their initiation and communication skills to help the injured as much as possible.

Be a Team Player

As pivotal it is to be a great leader, it is equally essential to be a team player. A first aider must, at all times, be cooperative, be it with fellow first aiders, the police or the emergency services.

Roles and Responsibilities of a First Aider

A first aider has several roles and responsibilities. It is vital that any first aider, whether certified or non-certified, fulfill these roles to the best of their capabilities as fulfilling them could potentially be lifesaving for someone. Other than providing the injured immediate medical care, the following are also the roles of a first aider:

- Performing CPR

- Placing the injured in a recovery position

- Using AED

- Keeping a spinal injury patient steady

- Stopping any external bleeding using elevation and pressure techniques

Other than these important roles, the first aider must also ensure that the condition of the injured doesn't worsen. The goal should be to promote recovery and help the patient get comfortable as opposed to just waiting on the medical experts to take over. Coming to the responsibilities of a first aider, they are as follows:

- Management of the incident while ensuring their safety and that of the injured and bystanders.

- Inquire about the nature of the injury and get as much information as possible (medical history, allergies, severe health conditions, etc.) out of the victim to help the medical experts.

- If there is more than one causality, prioritize administering first aid to those who are the most injured.

- If given the chance, take notes about how you found the patient, what caused the injury, what procedure you administered and any other important observations about the behaviors and symptoms of the casualties.

- Arrange for any other local emergency service if required. For example, the fire department in case of a fire.

- Fill out the paperwork and hand it over to the medical assistance upon arrival.

First Aid Myths and Common Mistakes

Several myths revolve around giving the first-aid wrong. Since it could be a matter of life and death, if you are the one administering it or seeing someone doing it wrong, it is your job to rectify so that more harm can be prevented. As you continue reading, you will be surprised how common it is for someone to respond with wrong first aid in cases of medical emergencies. To avoid making these mistakes, we are also going to tell you what you need to do instead.

Myth – If someone has swallowed something poisonous, make them vomit

It is best not to do so, especially if the patient doesn't complain of any irritation in their airways. A lot of times, when kids or adults swallow or drink poisons like bleach, asking them to vomit it out can cause further damage as the content has now been mixed with stomach acid and may react differently. Thus, there is an increased likelihood of it irritating the airways on its way back up when vomited. The same applies to any toy that has been ingested. If it didn't block the airways going down, it can block it on its way back up, which can cause severe breathing issues and cause choking.

So, what should be your approach?

Call for help and ask them how to proceed further. It also depends on how the patient is acting. Is he/she showing any signs of discomfort, complain of a burning sensation, etc.? Each situation will be treated differently, so try not to act hastily.

Myth – Ask someone having a heart attack to cough

Although many believe it to be the right thing to do and it has helped many people, but there is no medical evidence as to why it helps. This may allow a fresh flow of oxygen to the heart; it is still only a temporary way to manage a heart attack. This shouldn't be the only response to it. If one experiences chest pains, an ECG must be scheduled early to identify the root cause. A heart attack, like an earthquake, can have an aftershock and thus giving proper care the first time can prevent it from happening again.

Myth – You should scrape off a bee stinger

It is one of the most common mistakes people make when stung by a bee. The stinger must indeed be removed, but it has to be done right away and not later. The sooner it is scraped off, the better. Don't waste time by flicking it, brushing it or gently digging through it. The sooner it is done, the better and less painful.

Myth – Suck out the venom from a poisonous snake bite

Although 99% of snakes don't bite intentionally and are poison-free, in the event where one has been bitten by a poisonous snake, it is advised not to cut and suck the venom out like shown in most movies and shows repeatedly. Here's what experts believe: The venom doesn't just sit in one place. As soon as one is bitten, it runs through the bloodstream, causing clots along the way. Secondly, trying to suck it out is only a treat for the snake that bit as it now has two victims suffering from the same bite.

What should you do instead?

Use the pressure immobilization technique (PIT) to keep the venom from entering the bloodstream.

Myth – You must give a choking victim the Heimlich maneuver

Again, although presented as something easy for anyone to perform, there are documented cases of complications due to the Heimlich maneuver. It must only be performed when there is a complete blockage of the airways and the person starts to turn blue or becomes unable to speak. If that isn't the case, simply coughing it out can help. Since there are multiple delicate organs around the stomach region, when performed incorrectly, the Heimlich maneuver can cause life-long damage to the ribs and other vascularized organs.

Myth – You must blow into a bag when hyperventilating

There are hundreds of reasons that can get your heart beating faster. Exercise, excessive stress, anxiety, excitement and even love at times can leave you breathless. Breathing into a paper bag does no good in any of these conditions. Besides, it isn't even a proper treatment. The point being, it isn't going to make your stress or anxiety go away and you might want to see a doctor for that.

Myth – You must never move a person with spinal injury

Although this is the most ideal especially when you or the patient is unaware of the severity of the damage done. Moving them might only add to their discomfort and level of pain. But not moving them at all isn't right either. In some cases, where further danger is expected, the patient must be removed from the scene and carried onto one that is safe. If the patient isn't responsive or vomiting, it is best to lay them down in a resting position until help arrives.

Myth – If someone has been stung by a jellyfish, pee on them

Isn't that making beach vacations with kids weird 101?

True, peeing on a sting does work but only if the urine is acidic. You might as well use water instead of urine if it is diluted or less acidic. Since acidity is what matters, try carrying a bottle of vinegar the next time you go to the beach. It surely is going to work!

Myth – If a kid has something in their mouth, put your finger to remove it

Not only can your finger further push down whatever is it they have got stuck in their throat, but it can also lead to choking and blockage of the airways. For any parent or even a first aider, this will be an absolute nightmare.

So, what should you do instead?

If any foreign object has been stuck, use abdominal thrusts or back slaps to remove the blockage.

Myth – If someone is having a seizure, put something in their mouth to bite onto

Seizures are scary but they don't generally do much harm. Think of them as a way used by your body to communicate something's not right. They aren't themselves a condition but rather an indication of an underlying one. Now that we have that cleared, trying to insert something in a seizing patient's mouth isn't going to stop it. It can get stuck in their airway and block it. So, no need to stuff your wallet, a piece of cloth or any other non-sterile thing into their mouth and wait for help.

Myth – You should apply butter to soothe a burn

Butter may be the one thing easiest to grab from your pantry or a departmental store to ease the burning sensation, but it isn't going to help you or your doctor. If anything, it is only going to make the application of your medication harder. A burnt area is highly sensitive and to put something as non-sterile as butter on it can make it prone to infection. If someone has suffered a first-degree burn, it may be best to just pack it with some ice to allow healing or run under cold water. If it is a second or third-degree burn and involves swelling, blistering and intense pain, then only a certified physician must look at it and prescribe the best course of treatment.

Myth – You must put a steak on a bruised eye

If you have been doing this, it is time we correct you. It isn't the steak that does anything but rather the cold. Putting a steak that isn't frozen can introduce bacteria into the eye which can easily result in an infection. The goal is to apply something frozen to the eye to ease the inflammation and help the flow of blood. If you don't have a stake in your freezer, the same results can be achieved with a bag of frozen veggies or an ice pack.

Myth – If someone has a sprained ankle, apply a hot compress

Applying heat only worsens the tissues by adding to the inflammation. If anything, apply a cold compress to combat swelling and prevent it from worsening. A cold compress should be applied for 10 minutes as the first response and then later continued if the swelling doesn't go down. In case of a severe sprain or fracture, you mustn't apply anything unless the medical experts tell you to.

Myth – If you have a nosebleed, tilt your head backward

This is mostly the first response of parents and P.T. teachers. If only they knew how wrong it was. Did you know that leaning back when having a nosebleed can make you swallow the blood? And since the stomach isn't used to you drinking your blood or anyone else's, it is going to vomit it out which will only make matters worse. First, you only had a nosebleed and now you are also vomiting your guts out.

So, what should you do instead?

Lean forward instead. The blood that is already in your nose will run out anyway, thanks to gravity. Let it flow out and whilst doing that, place an icepack on your nose or head to stop the bleeding.

Myth – You should rub alcohol on someone with a fever

Wrong again! Alcohol, in general, has a cooling tendency. Rubbing alcohol or drinking it to warm up your body can do nasty things upon drying up. Look for other means to reduce your fever, such as placing a cold compress on the forehead and the soles of the feet.

Myth – You must never use a tourniquet

Although they have a bad reputation with first aiders and considered to cause irreplaceable harm in some cases, if it is a must, there isn't anything better than that. However, there are only a few acceptable conditions where it should be the first choice of a first aider. The first response, however, must still be the application of direct pressure to stop the bleeding.

Chapter 2
First Aid Kit Essentials

"It's also selfish because it makes you feel good when you help others. I've been helped by acts of kindness from strangers. That's why we're here, after all, to help others."

~ Carol Burnett

In this chapter, we are going to help you prepare your first-ever first aid kit. Although there are many different emergency kits for different situations, having basic know-how about some of them and how they must be used can be extremely helpful.

A Basic First Aid Kit

A basic first aid kit includes a collection of equipment and supplies essential to administering first aid. A first aid kit can vary in supplies and equipment based on the environment it is meant to use for home, outdoors, work, etc. Even in those categories, you may find subdivisions like the home kit can be for children, seniors, or disasters. The wilderness kit can be for camping, military or road trips/flights. Despite these differences, each kit has some particulars which include the following items listed below.

First Aid Manual

This is the most important essential of any basic first aid kit. A first aid manual lists how one can treat several health conditions and injuries such as wounds, bleeding, burns, stings, bites, etc. It also contains techniques on how to perform emergency procedures such as CPR, Heimlich maneuver, dressing bandages. Thus, it can prove to be extremely helpful in times of crisis.

Antiseptic Wash

An ideal situation would include cleaning the injured person's wound with water and soap. However, you won't always have a faucet available hence the antiseptic wash. An antiseptic wash comes out squirting in a thin but powerful stream to get rid of any dirt particles from a wound.

Tweezers

No matter how basic your first aid kit is, chances are tweezers will come in handy. This multipurpose tool can help hold the wound open, remove debris from the wound and also pick out any splinters. These also come in handy when you need to scrape off any stingers left behind.

Alcohol Swabs

Similar to an antiseptic wash, alcohol swabs help clean the wound before any ointment is applied or the area is bandaged. Alcohol prevents any formation of bacteria which eliminates the chances of an infection. Other than that, they can also be used as a sterilizing tool to clean scissors or tweezers.

Scissors

The next important thing in your first aid kit is a pair of good medical scissors as you are going to be cutting more than one adhesive bandage in case of a medical emergency. They can also help you cut with precision and trim any unwanted threads from bandages. When the removal of clothes is an absolute must, they can get the job done without any tears. Besides, a pair of medical scissors are easy to manipulate and safer than regular scissors.

Antibiotic Ointment

Antibiotic ointment, as the name suggests, is used for multiple purposes, such as cleaning the wound or helping it to heal quickly. Its primary function is to protect the wound from becoming infected. Its application must be repeated with every new bandage or stitches so that the wound remains clean.

Bandages

Adhesive bandages are one of the most pivotal supplies in any first aid kit. They come in different shapes and sizes to cater to different injuries. It is best to keep an assorted box of adhesive bandages in your first aid kit as you never know how big or how many you are going to need. As a general rule of thumb, you must have at least five in sizes small, medium and large.

Medical Tape

Medical tape, like regular tape, does the function of securing wounds when bandaged with wraps or gauze pads. Since gauze pads may be difficult to secure on their own, medical tape ensures the safety of the wound, preventing any dirt or debris from passing through.

Gauze Pads

Gauze pads are much bigger than adhesive bandages and also stronger in their hold. Since not all big wounds and cuts may be covered by an adhesive bandage, this is where a gauze pad comes in. They can be used as a bandage itself or as an absorbing pad to absorb blood and other bodily fluids. Like adhesive bandages, they too come in various sizes and having at least one of each is ideal.

Bite and Sting Treatment

Bites and stings are some of the most common injuries that people get. If not treated immediately, the sting can be extremely painful and even limit the blood flow to the injured area leading to swelling. Therefore, it is best to have ointments available that can ease the pain and swelling, especially when you live in warmer regions. In addition to the ointment, also have a small bottle of lotion or anti-bacterial cream to calm down any itching and redness from the area of the bite or sting.

Elastic Bandages

Elastic bandages are used to keep in place any sprained joints or ankles. The elasticity stops the area from becoming swollen and also prevents movement which may cause the injured person discomfort and pain. They have multipurpose uses as they can be used to hold in place the joints of knees, ankles, elbows and even shoulders. They come in various widths ranging from one to six inches.

Pain Relievers

Pain relievers shouldn't only be a part of your first aid kit but also essential in your bag that you take everywhere. They work wonders to help relieve the pain of any open wounds as well as for minor aches and pain.

Disposable Gloves

Disposable gloves come in handy (literally) when administering first aid to the injured. Not only do they protect your hands from bodily fluids, but they also help the injured by ensuring the affected area remains clean of any bacteria or microbes. Once you are done patching up the patient, the same gloves can be used to clean the surface where any blood or bodily fluids were spilled.

Instant Cold Pack

Cold packs are ideal to treat swelling and sprain-related injuries. Their application helps decrease the inflammation of the tissues or the muscles, relieve pain and discomfort. They come in sealed packages and are a one-time use product. They become icy cold when the seal from the packaging is opened and the material is activated.

Types of First Aid Kits

Home First Aid Kits

Home first aid kits are for all the people in your home. They come in handy whenever there is a medical emergency such as cuts, bruises, body aches or bug bites. A home kit must be stored in a safe but easy to access area in your house, such as a bathroom cupboard or kitchen cabinet. However, if there are children in the house, you might want to keep it in a place they can't reach easily. Be sure to do a bi-yearly check on all the medications and bandages to check for expiration dates.

Your Home First Aid Kit Checklist

Here is a list of all the essential items your home first aid kit must have:

- ❏ Adhesive bandages

- ❏ Adhesive tape
- ❏ Ace bandages
- ❏ Gauge pads
- ❏ Antiseptic lotion
- ❏ Pain relievers
- ❏ Scissors
- ❏ Tweezers
- ❏ Oral antihistamine
- ❏ Disposable gloves
- ❏ Safety pins
- ❏ Triangular bandages
- ❏ Pocket mask for CPR
- ❏ First aid manual
- ❏ Medical history of all the people in the house
- ❏ Emergency contact numbers and names of family members and relatives

Travel First Aid Kits

Travel kits are on-the-go first aid kits placed in your car or in the bag you are carrying when traveling abroad. A travel kit is equally as important as a home first aid kit, as you can never know when you will meet with an accident or calamity. Road accidents are the most common injuries brought to a hospital. Therefore, if you happen to find someone in need of first aid, your little medical box is going to come in handy and help relieve some of the stress from the situation until help arrives.

Your Travel First Aid Kit Checklist

The items in your travel first aid kit may vary depending on where you are going, the remoteness of the destination, the activity you are undertaking and for how long you will be gone. As a general rule of thumb, these are some of the essentials you must carry to help yourself and others in case of a medical emergency:

- Pain relief medication
- Antihistamine pills for allergies, bites or stings
- Cough medication
- Cold and flu medication
- Throat drops or lozenges
- Motion sickness medicine
- Antiseptic solution and ointments to clean and apply to an open wound
- Insect repellent
- Scissors

First Aid for Beginners

- ❏ Safety pins
- ❏ Sticking plaster
- ❏ Blister and wound patches
- ❏ Medical adhesive
- ❏ Diarrhea medicine
- ❏ Sting relief medication
- ❏ Antacid
- ❏ Antibacterial and antifungal cream
- ❏ Laxative for constipation
- ❏ Eye lubricant drops
- ❏ Sunscreen
- ❏ Health Insurance Card
- ❏ Thermometer
- ❏ Earplugs
- ❏ Spare pair of prescription glasses
- ❏ Mosquito-proof netting
- ❏ Hand sanitizer
- ❏ Water purifier tablets

- ❏ Prescription medications
- ❏ First aid manual

Office First Aid Kits

Although workplaces have to comply with many safety rules and regulations, accidents can still happen. Someone might take a bad fall, injure themselves by colliding with the corners of the desk or get paper cuts. Other than that, there are many other accidents just waiting to happen, such as a stuck elevator, fire or electrical short circuits. Before medical help arrives, everyone is on their own. Luckily with a first aid kit and a certified first aider, accidents will seem less stressful.

Your Office First Aid Kit Checklist

The workplace first aid kit is also essential. Before we reveal these, remember that the location of your business and what it deals with must also be taken into account. For instance, if you work surrounded by hazardous chemicals, you must have protective masks and gloves available at all times. You must also have burn ointment readily available to help someone in need immediately. Similarly, if your business is located in a desert/forest-based area, keeping anti-venom serums for snake bites or bug bites will help in case of an emergency. Although, the administration must arrange for one if you think of keeping a spare at hand, here is a list of things you are going to need in your kit.

- ❏ Gauze pads
- ❏ Gauze roller bandages
- ❏ Box adhesive bandages

- ❏ Triangular bandages
- ❏ Scissors
- ❏ Wound cleaning supplies
- ❏ Resuscitation equipment
- ❏ Tweezers
- ❏ Latex gloves
- ❏ Elastic wraps
- ❏ Blanket
- ❏ Disposable gloves
- ❏ Splint
- ❏ Protective mask
- ❏ Adhesive tape

Camping First Aid Kits

Imagine you are enjoying some time away from your work with your family in the wilderness. The kids are running up and down the stream collecting stones. Life looks good and carefree until one of them falls onto the ground and suffers a bad cut. There is blood gushing out and you are running here and there, grabbing pieces of clothing to cover and apply pressure to it. The cloth, if not clean, can cause bacteria and infection. Imagine if you just had a first aid kit with some adhesive bandages and antiseptic and antibacterial ointment and some pain relievers to help with the pain. Wouldn't the situation be much more in your control?

Your Camping First Aid Kit Checklist

If this has you convinced and you have decided to DIY a first aid kit for camping, here is the list of items you will need.

- ❏ Adhesive bandages of multiple sizes
- ❏ Gauze pads and rolls
- ❏ Butterfly bandages
- ❏ Antiseptic ointment
- ❏ Cleaning solution
- ❏ Sterile wipes
- ❏ Pain medicine
- ❏ Tweezers
- ❏ Safety pins
- ❏ Scissors
- ❏ Knife
- ❏ Sunburn relief spray
- ❏ Diarrhea medicine
- ❏ Antihistamine for allergies

- ❏ Moleskin
- ❏ Duct tape
- ❏ Eye drops
- ❏ Triple antibiotic ointment
- ❏ Hand sanitizer
- ❏ SPF cream
- ❏ Superglue
- ❏ Aloe Vera
- ❏ Emergency blanket

Disaster First Aid Kits

There are times when you might be told to stay indoors for several days or to leave your house and stay in a temporary shelter built by the government. This is very common in areas mostly facing war or severe weather conditions. Another reason why states suggest building a disaster first aid kit is that one may never know how long a natural disaster will last. If we just take wildfires, floods, tsunamis or heavy rain or snowfall as examples, you might better understand the need for a first aid kit. There have been cases where help from the local authorities was postponed for weeks and the survivors had to make it on their own. How would you feel if you were left with no food, water, or basic survival supplies and a family to care for?

Therefore, having a disaster first aid kit can't be stressed enough.

Your Disaster First Aid Kit Checklist

Here's a list of items your disaster first aid kit should include before utilities are restored and everything is back like it used to be.

- ❏ Food supply for three days (non-perishable foods)
- ❏ One gallon of water per person
- ❏ Crockery (utensils, plates, and spoons)
- ❏ Trash bags
- ❏ A can opener
- ❏ Dish soap
- ❏ Prescription medication
- ❏ Flashlight
- ❏ First aid manual
- ❏ Batteries
- ❏ Radio
- ❏ Whistle
- ❏ Flare
- ❏ Match sticks
- ❏ Bedding

- ❏ Fire extinguisher
- ❏ A few pairs of clothes and shoes including undergarments (per person)
- ❏ Bedding
- ❏ Toiletries
- ❏ Scissors
- ❏ Pocket knife
- ❏ Water filter straws
- ❏ Rain gear
- ❏ Plastic wraps
- ❏ Surgical masks
- ❏ Cash
- ❏ Copies of important documents
- ❏ ID
- ❏ Basic tools (screwdrivers, hammer, crowbar, pliers, etc.)
- ❏ Permanent marker, paper, pen
- ❏ Emergency contact numbers
- ❏ Duffel or backpack

- ❏ Cell phone and charger
- ❏ Cooking tools (pan, spatula, spoon, etc.)
- ❏ Sunscreen
- ❏ Plastic bottles

Chapter 3
Recognizing Emergencies

We have a responsibility to help those around us and help others in need.

-Virginia Williams

An emergency is someone getting stuck in an elevator, a road accident, bad weather or even childbirth without assistance. There are countless emergencies and disasters just waiting to happen – completely unpredictable and unexpected. They may happen a minute from now as you are reading this or years later when a volcano erupts in your hometown. The point is how do you recognize when it's happening right now someplace near you? Of course, some signs allow you to recognize the depth of the situation and whether medical assistance is required right away or not. Of course, your kid getting an earache isn't an immediate emergency but someone having a seizure is and calls for immediate attention.

Luckily, in this chapter, we are going to help you to recognize a medical emergency – an emergency that requires immediate medical attention. We shall also learn of any warning signs that we must watch out for and let others know as well.

What Counts as a Medical Emergency?
Recognizing an emergency allows you to respond. There is a slight difference between an injury and a medical emergency. An injury could be any wound, burn or fracture, whereas a medical emergency is

someone having a heart attack or losing excessive blood. Here are some pointers on how to spot a medical emergency.

Listen for Any Unusual Sounds

Noise is the first thing that gets someone's attention. Be it a baby crying in the room next door or your neighbor's dog shouting in the yard because it sees someone new at the door. Long before you are even near the place of the accident, you hear unusual sounds.

Some sounds that indicate that there might be a medical emergency include:

- Crying out in distress or pain
- Screaming
- Yelling
- Calling for help
- Moaning

Other noises may include:

- Breaking of glass
- Screeching of tires
- Crashing of metal
- Collapsing of buildings
- Falling ladders
- Flight crashing

- Incoming flooding etc.

Look for any Unusual Sights

A lot of times, we disregard or miss a sight that signifies a medical emergency. Sometimes, we think of it as a mere inconvenience. Below are some examples to help you understand.

- A fallen chair
- A stalled car
- A spilled medicine container
- A man lying in an alley
- Overturned saucepan on the floor
- Heavy cartons scattered on the ground etc.

All these can mean that something life-threatening happened and someone might require medical assistance. For instance, an overturned pan on the floor could mean someone had their hand burnt, a man in an alley could mean that he was mugged, shot or had a stroke. Signs that make you ponder because they seem out of the norm must never be ignored.

Sense any Unusual Smell

We are accustomed to many different smells. The smell of petrol, the smell of smoke, the smell of burnt food in the kitchen. However, we only smell them for a certain period. For instance, we smell petrol when we are at the gas station. We don't smell it after we leave. We smell burnt food only until we turn off the stove and wash the pot. However, when such smells exceed a certain time limit and continue to linger in the air, it can mean a medical emergency. If they seem stronger than usual, say, the smell of smoke coming through your window for more than 10 minutes, it could very well mean fire nearby and thus, you must not wait for another second to leave and offer help. But keep in mind that you must protect yourself first. If you keep sensing the smell of petrol in your car, it might be leaking, and we have all seen how it ends in movies with the car blowing up. Thus, if something feels wrong, distance yourself from it at the earliest opportunity.

Notice any Unusual Behavioral Change

It might be impossible to judge whether a person is acting out or if the behavior is normal. There is a reason why traffic police officers have breathalyzers to judge whether a person is drunk or not. This becomes even tougher when you are trying to identify any behavioral changes in strangers. Despite that, several signs and symptoms indicate a medical emergency. For example, someone collapsing on the floor. Very obvious, no? You might not even have to look for it as chances are someone around the collapsed is going to shout for help. What we are most concerned about are signs that almost pass under the radar that even the patient doesn't interpret correctly. These include:

- Breathing problems (Someone might disregard it for suffocation or anxiety)

- Clearing the throat repeatedly (Thinking something is stuck in the airway but not sure)

- Clutching the chest (It could mean a heart attack, but the person may think of it as gastric reflux or shortness of breath)

- Hesitant or slurred speech (One might think they are just unable to utter a difficult word at first but as they become more disoriented, one might not even be able to make out help. It can happen due to many reasons such as choking or a seizure.)

- Irritable behavior (It can indicate trouble feeling comfortable or going through some unexplainable underlying condition.)

- Going pale, flushed or blue (Again, this can indicate many things such as airway blockage, drug overdose, poor blood circulation or oxygen to the heart, etc.)

- Excessive sweating (Sweating can be a symptom of heart attack too but not many know of that. Therefore, precipitation is often waived off as just the heat in the room or blamed on tightly fitted clothes.)

If you notice any of these signs that seem odd for, let's say, at an office dinner setting, know that someone needs a medical emergency. Go up to them and ask them if there is something that they need or whether they are feeling alright.

Warning Signs of a Medical Emergency

Once you are certain that something is wrong and medical assistance is required, dial your local emergency number right away to let them know there is an emergency. Below are conditions that are the definition of a medical emergency

- Unstoppable bleeding

- Road accident injuries like broken bones

- No pulse or breathing
- Choking and airway blockage
- Unconsciousness
- Electrical shock
- A seizure that doesn't stop for more than 3-4 minutes
- Chest pains
- Self-destructive behavior
- Drowning
- Asthmatic attack
- Stroke
- Poisoning
- Insect bite reactions
- Allergic reactions
- Unable to detect the source of bleeding etc.

When met with any of these situations, let the 911 operator know the details of who you are, who is the patient, how is he/she, where you are and what have you done to manage the situation. Don't hang up on the operator until given permission as he/she might make you go through a few checks before dispatching help. He/she might inquire about the condition of the patient, what happened to them, was it something they ate that caused it, was the casualty behaving oddly, medical history of the patient in case they are a friend or family member, etc.

Is it An Urgent Medical Emergency?

Urgent medical conditions refer to conditions that a healthcare provider must be informed about as soon as they reach the scene. Even if the patient isn't suffering from them at the moment, letting the first aid provider know of their condition might help with the course of treatment. For instance, if someone you know needs first aid and they reported similar symptoms a week ago, it is best to let the first aid provider know. Likewise, if they are allergic to something or have been trying a new medication that may or may not have something to do with their current state, it is still best to let the responder know. You might want to let the healthcare provider know if the following physical and behavioral changes that tell you they need urgent care:

Physical Changes

- Fever that is higher than 101 °F or continues to rise
- A rash that has lasted longer than a week or so
- Vomiting that has lasted for more than 24 hours
- Persistent diarrhea
- Upset stomach
- Abdominal cramps but no period
- Pain is one of both legs for hours
- Feeling suffocated

- Low blood sugar levels
- Infection at the injured area
- Limping or difficulty in moving
- Swelling
- Difficulty swallowing or sore throat etc.

Behavioral Changes

- Sleepiness
- Difficulty in waking up
- Holding abdomen
- Sudden incontinence onset
- Dramatic facial expression changes
- Change in demeanor
- Scratching of one or both ears
- Depicting a self-injurious behavior
- Signs of some discomfort or pain

A Short message from the Author:

Hey, are you enjoying the book? I'd love to hear your thoughts!

Many readers do not know how hard reviews are to come by, and how much they help an author.

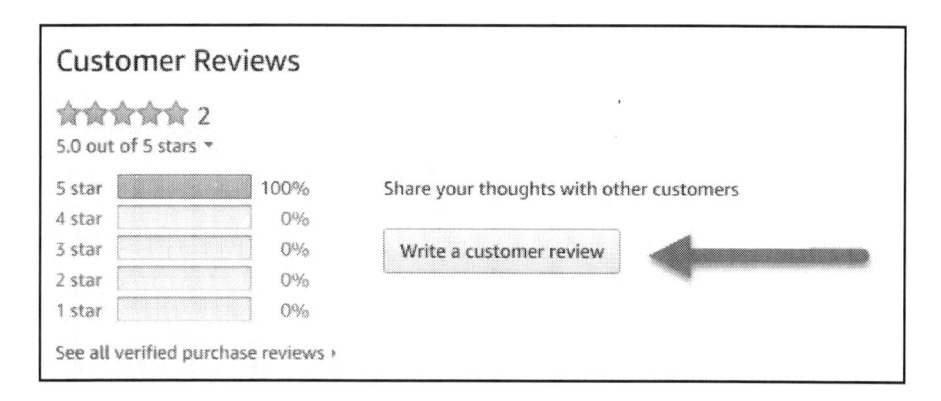

> **Customer Reviews**
>
> ★★★★★ 2
> 5.0 out of 5 stars ▼
>
> | 5 star | 100% |
> | 4 star | 0% |
> | 3 star | 0% |
> | 2 star | 0% |
> | 1 star | 0% |
>
> See all verified purchase reviews ›
>
> Share your thoughts with other customers
>
> [Write a customer review]

I would be incredibly grateful if you could take just 60 seconds to write a brief review on Amazon, even if it's just a few sentences!

\>\> Click here to leave a quick review

https://www.amazon.com/review/create-review?asin=B084DHDQWN

Thank you for taking the time to share your thoughts!

Your review will genuinely make a difference for me and help gain exposure for my work.

Chapter 4
Providing First Aid around Infectious Diseases

Somewhere along the way, we must learn that there is nothing greater than to do something for others.

~Martin Luther King Jr.

Infectious or contaminated spaces not only add to one's risk of attaining diseases and infections, but it also makes administering first aid without protective gear almost impossible. One must never approach a scene such as a burning fire or a chemical spill without protective gear as doing so could mean putting your own life at risk. And what help would you be to others if you are yourself for air as the smoke or infectious gases fill your lungs?

Therefore, to stress the importance of protective gear, we have dedicated a whole chapter to what you need and how you must approach spaces with contamination and how to proceed with caution and care.

Precautionary Gear Essentials

You can never know what you are getting yourself into when offering first aid to someone. Realistically, there are two types of danger – environmental and human danger.

1. Environmental dangers refer to any danger in the surroundings

such as broken pieces of glass, spilled chemicals, hazardous fumes or a collapsing structure.

2. Human danger, on the other hand, refers to any danger from the people in the area. It can be an oncoming vehicle at the scene of a car accident or the transmission of any blood-related diseases from the injured.

Thus, ensuring your safety against these two should be your priority. Here are some of the protective barriers you must always have on hand when dealing with injured people.

Gloves

To avoid any risk of disease transmission, you must always wear disposable gloves. They must be made of high-quality material and impermeable. Gloves prevent direct contact between the first aider and the injured and can protect you against any skin-related conditions and contagious infections.

There are typically three types of gloves available in first aid kits. These include:

1. Latex Gloves
2. Nitrile Gloves
3. Vinyl Gloves

CPR Adjunct

The next important protective essential that you need is a CPR adjunct, in case the patient isn't responsive and requires artificial resuscitation using mouth-to-mouth. With mouth-to-mouth, there is a greater chance of exchange and transmission of bodily fluids as you come near the patient. Sometimes, the stomach contents can also rise, leading to vomit, which you certainly want to stay away from. Luckily, with a CPR adjunct, you can maintain a safe distance as well as provide the patient with the help they require.

Other essential but optional equipment includes:

- Safety glasses (For workplace first aid)
- Gown or an apron
- Filter breaking mask

The Risks

In this next section, we shall look at various potentially hazardous situations where protection is a must and learn how to minimize the risk of acquiring an infection or diseases when attending to an injured patient. They include:

- Exposure to infected and blood-borne diseases while attending to a patient. Coming in contact with a patient with HIV or hepatitis B can be life-threatening to you as they are contagious and non-reversible. Thus, if the patient is responsive and you don't have protective gloves or an apron, ask them about any health conditions they might have and see if you are at risk of developing them as well in case you render them first aid. However, this transmission is only possible, if the first aider too is bleeding or has an open cut or wound on their body. Otherwise, there is very little chance, but it is best to be cautious.

- Exposure to alimentary tract infections in case the patient suffers from conditions like dysentery, salmonellosis or hepatitis A. If the patient has vomited and you are attending to them without protective gear, you may end up with one too. It happens rarely but there is still a possibility and as a healthcare provider you also must ensure your safety.

- Exposure to respiratory conditions and infections like brucellosis or tuberculosis when giving mouth-to-mouth CPR. The infection may travel their aerosol and enter your system without you even noticing. The tiny particles can travel into your mouth when you inhale.

Precautions to Take Around the Patient

As discussed before, you must think about your safety first then of others. Remember, if your gut tells you that the situation is going to get worse, take refuge first. For instance, if someone around you has been shot and there is a chance that more shots may be fired, instead of helping the injured, you must get to safety first and dial 911. Dialing 911 and alerting them of the situation is the best way to help the injured and yourself. Below is a list of some key points that you must remember at all times and try not to be a hero when your own life can be at stake. You will be no good to anyone else if you are injured yourself.

- Worry about your safety first and leave the scene if your life is at risk.

- When helping any victim, be sure to wear protective gear so that you may avoid transmission of infections and other diseases.

- Always have with you preventive breathing equipment when entering hazardous places.

- Before attending to the victim, cover your wounds, sores, cuts or skin conditions using a bandage.

- Don't attend directly with bare hands to bodily fluids and blood. Always use disposable gloves for protection.

- Before attending the patient, thoroughly wash your hands. Do the same after administering first aid to the patient.

- Let the injured remain in a steady position if you suspect any spinal or neck injury. Any sudden or unnecessary moves can worsen their condition.

- Always store your local emergency numbers including poison control, physician, and fire department on your phone.

Disinfection of Contaminated Areas

How do you clean up an area that has been contaminated with bodily fluids and blood? This is another imperative question that a first aider or healthcare provider must attend to before leaving the area. There are many reasons to ensure that the area where the injured was placed is disinfected. There is a possibility that if left contaminated, it can become a breeding ground for infections and disease-causing insects such as dengue-carrying mosquitoes or flies carrying infections and bacteria. The disinfection becomes even more important when space is used by others regularly such as the footpath or a bench in the park. So how do you go about disinfecting a contaminated are? Follow the steps below:

First Aid for Beginners

- First things first, before touching anything barehanded, wear protective gloves and preferably a mask as well to avoid coming in contact with the infection.

- Next, if the place is crowded (bystanders curious to know what you will do next), politely ask them to leave the space as it has been contaminated and must be cleaned for people to use it again.

- You must deal with any spillage immediately meaning, don't allow it to set in or dry up. It will only make the process of disinfection harder.

- If there are some blood splashes, use a paper towel or wet dressing to clean it. You may want to dampen the paper towel or dressing with an antiseptic and anti-bacterial solution. Disinfect the area at least twice before washing it with running water to ensure proper disinfection. Place the used towels or dressing pads in a plastic bag before disposing of them in a bin or disposal.

- If there is a large spillage of bodily fluid, you must use sand, cat litter or vermiculite to absorb/clean the area. Use loads of disinfectant solution once you have covered the area with sand or vermiculite. Let the disinfectant work its magic for at least 30 minutes before scoping the sand into a bucket. If you can still smell the odor or feel that the place needs another round of disinfectant, do it. Dampen paper towels with the disinfectant and then lay them on the area of spillage. Don't remove them until semi-dry and then run water over the area.

Precautions for Dealing with Body Fluids Spillages

The next big question is how will a first aider proceed if there have been some bodily fluids spillage? What will be the course of action, considering it may contain some blood-borne disease?

The following precautions must be taken by the first aider when there has been a casualty that has bled out. The reason you might want to be conscious is that some people (the injured) may not be aware of the diseases they are carrying. So even if you ask them and they tell you that they don't carry any such diseases, remember that prevention is better than cure.

- Firstly, check for any cuts or abrasions on your own hands or arms. If there are any, cover them up with waterproof dressings before proceeding to administer first aid.

- Ideally, your hands should be clean, i.e. thoroughly washed with soap and water before you render any help to the patient.

- If there is a large quantity of blood or bodily fluid that needs cleaning, covering your body with an additional layer of protection is recommended. You must wear disposable aprons when cleaning the affected area.

- In case there has been a splash onto your face or body, wash it off immediately with a soapy solution. In case the splash has entered your eye, you might want to irrigate it with running water or an eye disinfectant.

- If your clothes have come in contact with bodily fluids, they must be sent off to laundering or dry cleaning after you have washed off the blood with water and washing detergent. In case the splashes are big and gross, you might want to dispose of it. Be sure to place it in a sealed bag and label contaminated material so that no one else comes in contact with it either.

- After you have cleaned the area or attended the patient needing medical assistance, discard the gloves and aprons into a dustbin.

- Thoroughly wash your hands with soap and water and use a hand sanitizer once you are done.

Chapter 5
First Aid Techniques 101

You need an attitude of service. You're not just serving yourself. You help others to grow up and you grow with them.

~David Green

Similar to the techniques discussed in the previous chapter, there are also some other basic techniques that a first aider must know of and learn to perform. Since it can only take a minute for any situation to worsen, knowing these will give the first aider an upper hand to act quickly and save the patient's condition from worsening further. For instance, a patient choking can have a cardiac arrest if the airway remains blocked. Will the first aider let the patient suffer and not do something about it? No, he/she will have to perform CPR right away in case the casualty is unresponsive or not breathing at all.

Thus, until help arrives, it is their job to administer care to the patient in need. Learning these techniques will help you if you are the one rendering first aid to someone.

Using a Defibrillator (AED)

Defibrillators are devices that emit an electrical shock to the heart to allow it to beat again. Think of it as an automated version of chest compressions with a higher rate of success in a life-threatening situation. It emits an electrical shock after assessing the pace of the heart's rhythm.

First Aid for Beginners

If you come across someone having a cardiac arrest or who has gone unresponsive, every minute you wait before performing CPR or using an Automated External Defibrillator reduces the chances of them surviving by 10% (Bon, 2018). This means that you will have to act quickly and not wait for help to arrive and take over the situation. In case you don't have an AED available, ask the 911 operator if there are any public access AEDs nearby. If there are and you have gotten a hold of one, follow the steps below to use it correctly.

- Turn it on by pressing the green button and following the instructions.

- Peel the sticky pads that come with it and remove the patient's shirt for the right placement of them. If there is someone with you, ask them to help take it off while you locate the position. The defibrillator comes with picture stickers that tell you exactly where you need to place the pads on the patient.

- Place the pads onto the chest as directed in the picture.

- Once you have the pads stuck, stop performing CPR. You mustn't touch the patient when the pads start to assess the patient's heartbeat. Your hand on the patient might hamper the results.

- Once the defibrillator has analyzed the patient's heart rhythm, it will determine if a shock is required or not. If it tells you that it is required, it will ask you to press the shock button located on the device. As soon as you press it, the device will release an electrical shock. You must ensure that no part of your body or anyone else's body is touching the patient when the shock is released.

- The device will then let you know that the shock has been administered and if you need to continue with CPR or not.

- If it does, continue with performing chest compressions and mouth to mouth resuscitation until you notice signs of life from the patient or have a steady heartbeat again.

- You can now remove the shock pads from the patient and turn off the device.

Note: In case the patient doesn't respond with the first attempt of shock, use the defibrillator to shock the patient again. Then continue with the steps of performing CPR.

Resuscitation

When you come across a patient that looks like they are sleeping but doesn't respond to any touch or sound, they are likely unconscious. Unresponsiveness or unconsciousness can last for a few seconds or longer durations. It is usually a sign of some serious health condition and thus, must be attended to immediately.

The treatment, however, to wake someone from unconsciousness is different for different age groups. But the technique is fairly simple and can be performed by a first aider confidently until help arrives. We are going to learn the steps to bring back someone to a conscious state using resuscitation.

Babies

It is fairly difficult to spot an unconscious baby as they don't normally faint or lose consciousness. This characteristic is mostly associated with adults. Babies too can sometimes lose consciousness. Since breathing is normal, it can easily be mistaken for sleep. However, if after trying to wake them up they still don't respond, check for any changes in their heart rhythm and call 911 ASAP.

Until help arrives, here are the steps you need to follow to the core to revive an unconscious baby.

Step 1: Look for any response

Start by gently flicking the soles of their feet or tapping their earlobe. These two spots are recommended by most physicians when trying to wake up an infant from sleep for feeding.

If they don't respond or depict any movements, they are likely unconscious.

Step 2: Clear the airway

Gently tilt the head of the infant backward using your hand. Place one finger of your other hand on their chin.

Step 3: Check for breathing

Notice if you hear them breathing or feel the little gush of air from their nostrils or mouth. Also, take note of their chest movements. Continue this for 10 seconds.

Step 4: Hold the baby in the recovery position

If you hear them breathing, hold their body in the recovery position. Slightly tilt their head back as you hold them in your arms like when you cradle them. This will help clear the airway in case something has been stuck in their throat. It will also prevent them from breathing in their vomit or choking on their tongue.

Step 5: Start CPR if no breathing is felt

If the baby continues to breathe fine but still isn't responsive, wait for the medical experts to take over when they arrive.

In the meantime, if you think that the baby has stopped breathing, start CPR. Use gentle chest compressions by applying pressure onto their chests. If that doesn't work, give them mouth-to-mouth resuscitation. Continue until help arrives.

Children and Adults

Do you think a child or adult is acting unresponsive? If so, here is what you need to do to ensure they continue to breathe until further assistance arrives.

Step 1: Clear the airway

The first step involves using your one hand to slighting tilt their head backward. To do so, place your hand on their forehead and push it back gently.

Using the index finger of your other hand, open their mouth by placing it on their chin and lifting it. This should open the mouth.

Step 2 - Check for breathing

Now, you need to move your face closer to their mouth and hear if they are breathing or not. You can also check for signs of breathing by placing one finger below their nostrils. You can also check for breathing by noticing their chest movement. If they seem to be breathing alright, place them in the recovery position if they are lying on their back or their side.

Step 3: Place the patient in a recovery position

However, if you suspect that the patient might have suffered a spinal injury, ensure that their neck remains still in one place when moving them into a recovery position. Instead of tilting their head backward, use the jaw thrust technique, which is as follows:

Place both your hands on either side of the face and use your fingertips to gently lift the jaw. You must ensure that the neck remains steady and the mouth remains open.

Now wait for help to arrive and in the meanwhile, keep checking if the person is still breathing or not.

Step 4: Perform CPR

If the patient still doesn't respond, start CPR right away.

CPR

Cardiopulmonary resuscitation or emergency breathing can save a life. Despite knowing all the steps, sometimes even the most experienced of first aiders can administer them incorrectly, which is why if you are just learning about it for the first time, keep a note of all the steps and complete them correctly. To help you administer CPR correctly, we shall guide you through each step in detail so that it can help you to help someone else.

However, before you begin administering CPR to anyone, there are several considerations you need to make. First being, how do you know if the patient requires CPR or not?

Here's how you may determine that:

- Shout "wake up" at the unresponsive patient. Call out their name if you know it.

- Hold them by the shoulders and shake them briskly. If they still don't respond, follow the next steps.

- Call 911. If a patient is breathing but is unresponsive, let the operator know that you are in dire need of the medical emergency unit.

- Look for signs of breathing. Place one hand on their forehead and use the index finger of the other hand and place it on the chin. Then tilt the head a little backward by putting pressure on the hand the forehead. This should open their mouths. Listen for breathing or sense it by placing a finger under the nostrils.

- If the patient doesn't breathe even after 10 seconds, begin CPR without wasting another second.

Performing CPR: The How-To

Step 1: Survey the Area

Is the area safe? Will you be able to reach the patient without any risks? This is the first thing you need to think about: your safety.

Step 2: Check for responsiveness

For an infant, tap the soles of their feet to check if they are responsive or not. You can also tap the earlobes. For adults, shake them by the shoulders vigorously and ask them aloud if they are okay. If you sense a reaction, they might not be unresponsive. If not, follow the steps below.

Step 3: Begin CPR

If the patient isn't responsive, start CPR right away, especially if it is a child or a patient who had drowned.

Step 4: Use an AED

With the help of an automated external defibrillator, look for any heartbeat or rhythm. Follow all the instructions listed on the machine from sticking the pads to administering the shock. If after the shock, the patient still isn't responsive, start chest compressions

Step 5: CPR technique

To perform CPR on an adult, use one of your hands and place it in the middle of the patient's chest. Then place your other hand on top of your firsthand and intertwine your fingers and draw them up. This will leave you with the palm of your firsthand directly in contact with the patient's chest.

If you are performing CPR on an infant, instead of placing your hand, just use two fingers instead. Place them in the middle of the chest between the nipples.

When performing CPR on toddlers or children, use only hand to perform chest compressions instead of two.

Step 6: Start chest compressions

When performing chest compressions on an adult, use your upper body's strength to build pressure. Start pushing onto their chest. You must perform 100 to 120 compressions per minute. Stop for a few seconds in between to allow their chest to recoil.

When performing chest compression on infants, release the pressure a little and give more recoil time to their chest in between compressions. Ideally, you should perform 80-100 chest compressions per minute.

In children, you must perform 100 to 120 chest compressions using the same technique used for adults.

Step 7: Continue compressions

Until help arrives or the patient begins to respond, continue performing CPR. If the patient starts to breathe normally, make them lay on their side and wait for the medical experts to arrive.

Dressing a Wound

A dressing keeps the wound clean and prevents against infection. A regular change of dressing can also speed up the process of healing. Ideally, a dressing should be big enough in size and width that it covers the whole of the wound with extra left around as a safety margin. Any basic first aid kit contains sterile dressings that are used to stop bleeding in deep wounds and soak up any discharge from a smaller wound like a whitehead or pus-filled blister.

During the administration of first aid, two types of dressings are used:

- Self-adhesive dressings
- Gauze dressings

The self-adhesive dressing is used to cover smaller wounds such as minor cuts and abrasions. There are multiple sizes and shapes to choose from, each serving a different purpose.

Gauze dressings, on the other hand, are thicker cotton pads used to cover bigger and deeper wounds. They are used to stop bleeding. Since they are thicker and heavier, an extra layer of protection (bandage or medical tape) is required to keep them in place.

If someone needs a dressing to cover a wound or cut, follow these steps below:

- Wash your hands thoroughly before coming in contact with the wound. If soap and water aren't available, use a hand sanitizer instead.

- Put on disposable gloves. If they aren't available, you should wrap your hands in a clean plastic bag or cloth. Using your bare hands to attend to the wound should be your last resort as you don't know what diseases the patient might carry.

- Once your safety towards the wound has been ensured, move onto administering first aid to the patient. The first step is to control the bleeding.

- You must get all bleeding under control before laying down the dressing. To do so, gently apply pressure onto the wound to squeeze out any blood. You should use a clean piece of cloth or a clean, dry bandage to clean the wound.

- Apply direct pressure on the wound to help form blood clots which will stop the bleeding. A large wound takes up to 20 minutes to form blood clots and stop bleeding, however, it may take you some more time depending on how deep the laceration is.

- If it continues to bleed after 20 to 30 minutes, you must take the patient to a hospital. The more blood loss, the harder it will become for the patient to respond or stay conscious. The delayed clotting of blood can indicate that the patient is on blood thinners or has some underlying clotting issues.

- If the bleeding has stopped, it is time to clean the wound. If there are any visible pieces of debris such as dirt, grass, or glass in the wound, use sterile tweezers to remove it. To sterilize the tweezers, dip them in rubbing alcohol to prevent the transfer of any bacteria or infection. Make sure you are gentle with the tweezers and not pushing in too deeply into the wound.

- In case you are finding it difficult to remove large pieces of debris or the patient complains of feeling too much pain, leave the removal and cleaning of the wound for the professionals. If by accident, you pulled out a piece of debris entangled with a blood vessel, it will start bleeding again.

- Medical experts suggest that it is best to rinse the wound first and then try to remove debris. This works in situations where there is little to no debris and you are just rinsing the wound for precautionary measures or when the debris is just some dirt or grime.

- If the wound is difficult to clean or bandage due to clothing, remove it or cut a section of it. This will help with the cleaning of the wound as well as dressing it after. If it is a woman wearing jewelry or accessories, remove that as well. This is an important step because in some cases, due to excessive bleeding, the area of the wound swells up. Thus, it is best to remove any piece of clothing or jewelry first. The same applies to any leg wound. If pants are hindering the process of dressing, then they must be removed or cut from around the area of the wound to provide better access.

- If the bleeding is still out of control, you might want to wrap the wound in a piece of cloth by making a tourniquet. However, they should only be used as a temporary covering as the tissues may start to die within a few hours without blood.

- Once clothing, accessories or jewelry have been removed, wash the wound with a saline solution to further clean it of any remaining debris or dirt. The saline solution works well as it contains bacterial properties. The action of rinsing sterilizes the wound.

- If there is no saline solution available, then rinse the wound with clean water. Hold the wound several times under water. The temperature of the water must be lukewarm or cold by never hot.

- Next, gently dab the wound with another piece of clean cloth using gentle pressure. The goal is to squeeze out the saline solution or water before applying the dressing. The act may allow some more bleeding to start but don't worry about that.

- The wound is not ready to be dressed. To help the dressing stick better and not adhere directly on the wound, apply an antibacterial cream to it. This will make it easier to change the dressing when needed as sticking to it directly may cause pain and bleeding when removed. An antibacterial cream will prevent infection as well as keep away any bacteria from entering the wound. If an antibacterial cream isn't available, you might want to use a hand sanitizer as it works similarly.

- Now place the dressing onto the wound and use a bandage, gauze pad or medical tape to wrap around it. Don't be too harsh with the wrapping as it may stop the circulation of blood. It should be tight enough that you can't stick your finger inside and loose enough that the skin around the wound doesn't swell up.

- Once you have dressed the wound, evaluate it. Note how long it stays dry. If you can see patches of blood on the bandage, it means the bleeding hasn't stopped. You might want to rush the patient to the ER to get those stitches right away.

Bandaging a Wound

Everyone should know how to bandage a wound and not just a first aider. Cuts, abrasions, and wounds can happen anywhere, even at home or at work. A simple paper cut to a deep laceration from a knife or tool can lead to unstoppable bleeding which must be prevented before too much blood is lost. Too much blood loss can lead to low blood pressure, resulting in the patient fainting or becoming unresponsive. But before we learn how to bandage, you must know of the available types so you can use the right one for a specific wound or cut.

There are three different types of bandages:

1. Roller

2. Triangular

3. Tubular

They are required when:

- An open wound needs covering

- A strained/sprained ankle or joint needs support

- Pressure needs to be applied to control or stop bleeding

Roller Bandages

Roller bandages are the most readily available type of bandage. They are a requisite in almost all first aid kits, even when there are no other types of bandages. They are multipurpose bandages and made from a continuous single strip of lightweight cotton. Since the strip is fairly thin, it must be wrapped several times around the wound to ensure the dressing underneath remains in its place and pressure is built on the wound.

Even a basic first aid kit will have a thick roll of roller bandages. They are primarily used to keep the dressing in place but due to their elasticated design, they also work great when a joint needs support. When used with a gauze pad, they can also help control bleeding which is one of the most important factors. They come in different sizes and thicknesses depending on how big or small of a wound needs to be covered. The thicker ones are more elastic, denser in the weave and can be used to cover big abrasions and cuts.

Triangular Bandages

Triangular bandages are versatile. They come with a single sheet of cotton or calico padding used to create slings to support soft tissue injuries, and to immobilize broken bones and fractures.

You can even use triangular bandages to improvise in an emergency. They can fashion a makeshift tourniquet. In case you are running short on roller bandages, you can use triangular bandages to wrap a dressing and tie two ends to keep a steady pressure until a doctor looks at the bones.

Some advanced first aid kits also come with triangular bandages with big safety pins to facilitate the process of sling construction.

Tubular Bandages

Tubular bandages aren't very ideal or versatile. They take the form of a tube when putting on a wound. They are designed to cater to just one body part at a time. They come in free size. The length, however, may vary. They are made from thick gauze and are used to provide compression. They are most ideal for supporting and immobilizing joints such as the knees, elbows, and ankles.

Steps to Bandaging

1. Start with finding the right bandage for the kind of wound you are catering to. Find one that hasn't been opened and is in the size you want. Ideally, a bandage should cover the dressing in one roll – meaning, it should be thick enough to cover the wound completely. If it is merely a small cut such as a paper cut, an adhesive band-aid would do the job.

2. If it is a larger wound, cover it with the dressing first cut into the right size and shape. While doing so, try to avoid any direct contact with the wound to avoid any inflectional risks.

First Aid for Beginners

Sometimes, with larger wounds, it is best to apply or lightly smear the open wound with an antibiotic cream. Not only will it deter any infection, but it will also hold the dressing better. Keep in mind that dressing a wound without an antibiotic cream will make it harder to pull off as the drained blood clots and stick to the wound like glue. Additionally, when it is removed, the wound may begin to bleed again.

3. After you have secured the dressing in place, use a non-stretch medical tape to further secure it. The tape should be cut longer than the size of the dressing so that it can stick to the sides of the skin. Be sure to secure the ends at a safe distance from the wound and onto a healthy piece of skin as you don't want the patient to feel additional pain when trying to take it off.

4. If you don't have medical tape on you and are thinking of securing the wound with industrial or electrician's tape, it is best to omit the tape completely. Since these tapes are designed to hold large appliances or wires together, they can tear the skin when pulled.

5. After you are done securing the wound, cover it up with an elastic roller or tubular bandage. However, you must ensure that you haven't wrapped it so tight that it hinders the blood circulation. It must only be tight enough to keep pressure built onto the wound to control the bleeding.

6. If required, secure the ends of the bandage with safety pins, metal clips or medical tape.

Notes:

- If there is a likelihood that the dressing will soon be damp, use a sheet of clear plastic between the dressing and the covering bandage to prevent the bandage from getting soaked. This additional layer will also prevent the formation or breeding of bacteria and other infectious agents.

- If the wound is on your head, shoulder or back, you might want to wrap it around your head, chest or waist to keep the wound from bleeding further.

- If the wound has been attended to by a physician and the patient has been told to leave and rest, it is important that the dressing on the wound is changed at home daily. A fresh dressing promotes the process of healing as well as keeps the wound clean. You can reuse the other bandage as long as it remains dry and hasn't been soaked.

- If you happen to spill water on your dressing for some reason (A splash of water, getting wet in the rain or mistakenly pouring water on the wounded area while taking a bath) don't wait for it to dry on its own or wait for another day to change it. A wet dressing promotes infection.

- Repeatedly check for any signs of infection as long as you keep dressing the wound. Sometimes, despite all your efforts, your skin might get infected or suffer from poor blood circulation which may form clots or leave your skin looking pale or bluish.

Other signs that indicate that there has been an infection include:

- Discharge

- Puss (yellowish or greenish)

- Pain and discomfort
- High fever
- The skin turning red
- Feeling sensitive upon touch
- Increased swelling

If you notice any of these, contact a doctor straight away. They might start you on some antibiotics right away. If the infection continues to grow, consider getting a tetanus shot.

Chapter 6
14 Basic First-Aid Procedures Everyone Should Know

"I think it's important, as a human being, to help others."

~Jason Derulo

There are a number of accidents that happen every day. You are at the beach and someone is stung by a jellyfish, you are calmly enjoying a Mexican tortilla and someone next to your table starts to choke, you are out shopping and someone collapses on the ground due to heatstroke, you are playing with your kids and accidentally hit your elbow against their nose causing a bleed, you are walking down the stairs and miss a step leading to a sprained ankle…

The point being, accidents can happen anywhere, to anyone and at any time. As a responsible citizen, it is your job to ensure that the people around you, be it your family members or complete strangers stay safe. In this chapter, we shall be looking at some of the most common accidents and medical emergencies that happen all the time. Are you prepared to tackle them on your own? If not, take a look below and learn about some of the easiest and manageable first aid procedures to help yourself and the people around you.

Cardiac Arrest

A cardiac arrest refers to a serious condition in which the heart stops pumping blood. Some of the most prominent signs that one is having a cardiac arrest include breathing problems and loss of consciousness. Since both of these conditions can be life-threatening if not attended to immediately, you must know how to perform cardiopulmonary resuscitation (CPR) instead of waiting for help to arrive.

Firstly, if you have a first aid kit on you with an automated external defibrillator, use that to check the heart's rhythm. If not, then call 911 right away and ask the operator if there is an AED for public access nearby. Luckily, if you can get your hands on one, it will make the situation less stressful and you will feel more in control of it. If not, you mustn't wait another second before starting with chest compressions and mouth-to-mouth resuscitation.

Even if you aren't trained to perform CPR, just remember that the goal is to allow the heart to start pumping blood again. Press hard and repeatedly, using your hands and upper body strength in the middle of the patient's chest. Try to aim for at least 100 chest compressions per minute. Stop in between to check if the heart is responding and breathing has been restored or not. Continue until medical help arrives. When they do, step aside and let them take over.

Choking

Choking is the result of airway blockage. It happens when something gets stuck in the throat or windpipe, limiting the intake of oxygen and the release of carbon dioxide. In infants or toddlers, a small piece of a toy or other object is usually the thing to blame. In adults, it is mostly chunks of food that get stuck in the windpipe, blocking air. Since it cuts off oxygen to the brain, if you notice someone choking, you must respond quickly.

Ask the patient choking whether they can cough it out or vomit the obstruction. If they aren't able to talk, are clenching their palms together or starting to turn red, it is a sign that the condition is serious. Although performing a Heimlich maneuver might seem the right thing to do as depicted in the movies, it should be the last resort, especially if you aren't trained to perform it.

Start by slapping their back to allow the obstruction to either pass down or come right back up. To do this:

- Stand behind or onto the side of the choking individual.

- Place one hand on their chest and motion them to bend forward. Their upper body should be parallel to the ground. Give them five blows onto their back in between the shoulder blades or lower using your other hand's heels.

- Don't remove your hand from their chest while giving them the blows. It might upset their balance and they might fall headfirst onto the ground.

If that doesn't work, try using the Heimlich maneuver, also referred to as the abdominal thrusts. Here's how you are going to perform the Heimlich maneuver:

- Stand behind the choking individual. For better support and grip over the patient, place one foot slightly forward than the other one.

- Wrap your arms around the choking individual's waist.

- Slightly tip the individual forward.

- Make a fist with one of the hands. Ideally, your fisted hand should be just above the naval.

- Your second hand should grip the fisted hand by the wrist.

- Using your upper body strength, press hard into the individual's stomach. It should be a quick, one-time upward thrust at first.

- When attempting the thrust, try lifting the individual from the ground.

- If the first attempt doesn't help in dislodging the blocked item, continue with the abdominal thrusts by increasing their number and intensity.

- You should perform six to nine abdominal thrusts to get the blocked item removed.

- In case that doesn't help, and the person starts to lose consciousness, lay him down on the ground and begin with CPR and rescue breathing.

- Continue with CPR until help arrives and then let them take over from there.

Sprains

Sprains aren't as alarming an injury as unresponsiveness or choking. In most cases, they heal on their own but might take a few days before the pain completely goes away. Sprained ankles or elbows result from falls, trips, and slips. They can be left untreated unless the area starts to swell. Swelling means that there is increased blood flow to the area which can either be due to tissue damage or injured vein. Whichever is the cause, the swelling must be reduced. Hot and cold compresses are often suggested by many to reduce swelling. Cold compresses are a much faster way to heal a sprain as it restricts the flow of blood by freezing the blood vessels which brings down the swelling.

In case someone has sprained their ankle, elbow or wrist, here's how you are going to help them feel better and ensure they haven't fractured a bone.

- Elevate the injured limb and place it on a steady surface.

- Apply ice to the area. Don't apply it directly to the skin but wrapped in a piece of cloth or a plastic bag.

- Compress the area gently with the ice. You can either hold it or fold the cloth or plastic bag with a bandage for steady support. However, be sure not to wrap the area so tight that it cuts off all circulation.

- Remove the ice pack after a few minutes and gently press down on the injured area to reduce the swelling.

- Continue alternating between compressions and the application of ice.

Frostbite

Frostbite happens when the tissues in our bodies freeze due to excessive exposure to cold. The area may become so numb that you might not even realize that it is frozen or feel any cut or abrasion into it. The formation of ice crystals into the tissues can lead to cell damage if left untreated. Think of it as a burn but only due to cold. Like any burn, whether major or minor, frostbite causes equal damage to the layers of the skin, the underlying tissues, and the cells.

One might think that the treatment for frostbite must be dipping the injured area into mildly hot water or putting hot compresses over it. It isn't! Medical experts strictly forbid the use of heating pads or any other form of heat to treat frostbite. Skin-to-skin contact is the best way to treat frostbite. But it must be done with extreme care and not in a hasty manner. The process of defrosting the injured area is a gradual one. A medical expert should be chosen to treat the frostbite and not just any individual.

Nosebleed

Nosebleeds are common among people of all ages. Sometimes they are a result of some direct injury to the nose such as a ball hitting you in the face or due to an upper respiratory infection or an obstruction. In kids, a small piece of toy or food like a pea or lentil getting stuck is one of the most common causes of nosebleeds. In adults, it is usually due to extreme picking of the nose, an injury to the nose or an allergic reaction.

Since they are so common, they are also easy to treat. You don't have to be a professional first aider to treat a nosebleed. But like any other procedure, there are a few steps you must follow to minimize the loss of blood.

- If you or someone has a nosebleed, ask them to lean forward instead of back.

- Next, pinch the nose from the bridge. Don't pinch the nostrils together as it will only restrict the blood flow and cause a blocked area.

- If the pinching doesn't work, apply a cold compress on the bridge of your nose or just below it to limit the blood flow by restricting the blood vessels.

- Keep the ice pack for about a minute or so and check if the bleeding has stopped or not.

- If the bleeding is the result of some direct thrust onto the nose, there is also a possibility that the individual might have broken a bone. In that case, it is best to take the patient to a hospital to get an MRI or X-ray done.

Allergic Reactions

Allergic reactions are a reaction from your body when it comes in contact with a substance that it rejects. Allergic reactions are fairly common across the globe. Some people are allergic to certain foods such as dairy or nuts while others are allergic to stings and drugs.

When an individual suffers from an allergic reaction, it can become life-threatening if it escalates to anaphylaxis. It is a severe condition after an allergic reaction which can cause the person's body to swell up. The airways and arteries swell up limiting the blood circulation and oxygen. This sudden decrease of oxygen and blood can result in breathing problems and even cardiac arrest. Thus, immediate help should be administered to the patient.

An EpiPen is the safest and fastest way to treat an allergic reaction. The epinephrine auto injector or EpiPen is an ergonomic needle filled with epinephrine. This small needle is injected into someone suffering from an allergic reaction. The epinephrine helps subdue the effects of the reaction. Below are some steps to administer first aid to an individual suffering from an allergic reaction.

- Tell the individual to remain calm and not panic. If they are allergic to something, chances are that they might carry an EpiPen with them. Ask them if they have it on them right now.

- If yes, tell the person to lie down on their back.

- Keep their feet elevated from about 12 inches from the ground.

- Loosen up any tight buttons and loosen their belt to allow them to breathe better.

- Don't give them anything to eat or drink, including medicine.

- Open the clear carrier tube to remove the EpiPen.

- Hold the EpiPen in your dominant hand and make a fist. Its orange pin must be pointing downwards. Ensure that your fingers aren't blocking either of the ends.

- Remove the blue safety release on one end of the EpiPen. It should come off easily.

- Position the person to receive the injection and let them know that you are going to inject them before doing it.

- Push the orange tip firmly into the upper thigh muscle. Keep pushing until you hear a clicking sound.

- Continue holding it for 3 more seconds before removing it.

- Gently massage the injected area for the next 10 seconds.

- Wait for 5 to 10 minutes to see if the symptoms of the allergic reaction subdue. If not, administer another shot using the same technique.

Don't administer more than two shots at a time. If the symptoms persist, it is best to call 911 and wait for further instructions from an expert.

Bee Sting

If someone is allergic to the venom, a bee sting can be both painful and deadly. In case someone has suffered from a sting, you must act quickly and prevent the sting from swelling. Below are some ways to treat a bee sting.

- First off, remove the stinger from the injured area to prevent further delivery of the venom into the bloodstream. One can use their bare hands to remove the stinger.

- In case the individual is allergic to bee stings, use an EpiPen to prevent him/her becoming anaphylactic.

- Call 911 for help and let them know about the condition of the injured.

- If the site starts to swell up, apply ice packs to prevent further swelling.

- To deal with the pain, the individual can take a pain reliever and an antibiotic to prevent itching and swelling.

Until help arrives, keep an eye out for any symptoms of anaphylaxis such as shortness of breath, itching in other body parts, redness or hives.

Heatstroke

Like frostbite, heatstroke occurs when someone spends a lot of time in the sun. The excessive exposure to high temperatures leads to dehydration via perspiration. This leaves the body feeling weak and dizzy. Other common signs of heatstroke include a weak pulse, muscle cramps, moist or cool skin, nausea, and headaches. Although, the symptoms may seem to subdue on their own when the person is moved to a cooler place like under shade or a facility, if left untreated, it can result in fatalities. In countries where temperatures go as high as 45 ℃, heatstroke is a leading cause of death during summers.

Thus, if you happen to notice someone depicting similar signs, here's how you need to act.

- First things first, take the person inside or under a shaded area where exposure to the sun is cut off.

- In case there is no such area nearby, cover the head and face of the individual with a piece of cloth or material. The goal should be to block sunlight.

- Give the person a lot of water to drink so that their body remains hydrated. You can also substitute water for a glass of fresh juices or flavored water to give an extra boost of vitamins and glucose.

- Place a damp piece of clothing on their forehead to lower their temperature.

If their condition continues to worsen and you sense a decline in their pulse or consciousness, call 911 and seek medical help.

Cuts and Scrapes

Our body usually heals any cuts and scrapes on its own. However, with deeper cuts that go deep into multiple layers of the skin, it becomes harder for the antibodies to patch it up. Deeper cuts and scrapes require medical attention to stop the bleeding as well as stitching it back up.

If someone has suffered a deep cut or abrasion, here is what you need to do.

- Your first goal is to stop the bleeding. To do so, apply pressure directly to the wound and not on its sides. Pressure on the wrong spot will only lead to further bleeding.

- If you have adhesive dressing or gauze pads on you, use those to cover the wound to limit exposure to infections and bacteria in the air. Don't apply any ointment without seeking medical advice first.

- Bandage the dressing with another piece of cloth to keep the pressure on the wound built. If a dressing isn't available, use another piece of cloth and make a tourniquet with it.

Bleeding

Almost all bleeding is controllable no matter how severe the injury. Mild bleeding usually stops on its own. For severe bleeding, you might need to act fast. The more someone loses blood, the higher their chances of going into shock or lose consciousness. This can also mean death. Follow these steps if someone has been badly injured and the bleeding is severe.

- Cover the injured area with a piece of cloth or dressing.

- Using your hand, apply direct pressure on the wound gently. Don't remove the cloth unless it has been drenched with blood. If that happens, use another clean cloth to cover the wet dressing. The dressing will help with the formation of blood clots which will help in stopping the flow.

- If you have a bandage on you, use it to cover the dressing and drive the patient to the hospital or call 911 for emergency medical services.

Fracture

Nearly all extremity injuries are treated as fractures unless an X-ray suggests otherwise. There is no sure way to tell whether a bone has been broken or dislodged from its original position. Of course, some people say they heard it click or crack but unless the area has been X-rayed there is no way to tell. This leaves first aiders to decide on their own how they are going to treat it. Are they going to treat it as a mild sprain, dislocation or a fracture? It is best to treat it as a fracture as the former two are less severe. Fractures, on the other hand, can be extremely painful and take months before healing completely.

Thus, if you suspect that someone has fractured a limb, here's what you need to do.

- Your instinct might tell you to straighten it, but don't; You might end up causing more damage to the bone.

- Start with trying to stabilize the fractured limb using padding and a splint. These two will help keep the limb immobile.

- If the area starts to swell up, use an icepack on the injured area. Don't put ice directly on the injured part as it may cause frostbite. Wrap it in a paper towel or a piece of cloth before applying.

- Next, elevate the extremity.

If the pain becomes unbearable, you may want to start the patient on some pain reliever or an anti-inflammatory drug such as naproxen or ibuprofen.

Blisters

Blisters are sacks filled with liquid that resemble a pimple. These usually happen due to friction between the body and clothing or from burning. But are they an emergency? It depends on how painful or uncomfortable they become. They require attention when they start to hinder one's daily routines such as experiencing pain while walking or being unable to perform simple tasks such as showering. If they aren't painful, they might as well be left to heal on their own. Just be sure to cover them so as to prevent pressure or further rubbing.

However, if it is large and causing you pain, here's what you need to do.

- Use a sterilized injection needle to puncture the bubble so that the pus or liquid inside drains out.

- Apply an antibiotic cream to prevent it from getting infected and cover it with dressing or an adhesive bandage to prevent further rubbing. It should dry out and heal after a few days. If needed, reapply the antibiotic ointment to help it heal faster.

Burns

Burns are of various kinds and categories. Therefore, before administering first aid to someone who has been burnt, you must analyze the extent and severity of the burn. Burns are classified into four different categories as follows.

- First-degree burns: In a first-degree burn, only the outer layer of the skin is burnt. It looks very similar to a sunburn or tan, only slightly swollen and red.

- Second-degree burn: In a second-degree burn, a few inner layers of the skin are burnt. It can cause swelling, blistering and is accompanied by extreme pain.

- Third-degree burn: In a third-degree burn, all the seven layers of the skin are burnt. The skin turns black or has a whitish color to it. Some burns can be so severe that even the nerve endings are destroyed. Due to this, the injured might experience no pain.

- Fourth-degree burn: In a fourth-degree burn, the injury penetrates the tissues up to the bones and tendons. It is the severest form of burn and the damage is irreversible.

Burns are also classified based on their severity such as minor or major.

Minor burns are first and mild second-degree burns whereas major burns are moderate second to severe fourth-degree burns.

To treat a minor burn, you must:

- Run the injured area under cool water.

- If there are blisters, don't try to break or puncture them.

- Next, you must apply a soothing ointment or moisturizer. An anti-inflammatory moisturizer containing Aloe Vera is best. Repeat the application several times a day to keep the area from drying out.

- Avoid going into the sun for a few days or until the burn has been healed. If going out is a necessity, cover the area with a piece of clothing.

- If the pain persists, you may want to give the person a pain relief medication.

Major burns require a trip to the hospital at the earliest opportunity and an examination by a doctor. The best you can do is prevent the application of any ointment as you don't know how much damage has been done. You also mustn't cover the wound with a tight bandage or dressing.

Jellyfish Stings

Jellyfish are known to sneak up on their victims and leave behind the most painful of marks and stings. If you are on the beach and someone has been stung by a jellyfish, follow these steps below to administer first aid.

- Rinse the area with something acidic like vinegar for at least 20 seconds. This should alleviate some of the pain. If you don't have vinegar, use a baking soda slurry instead.

- Next, you need to immerse the affected area in hot water. It shouldn't be burning hot but hot enough for the person to bear it. Let the injured area soak in the water for about 20 minutes or until they stop complaining about the pain. You can also use hot or cold packs if hot water isn't available. Don't bandage the stung area.

- If necessary, apply a soothing ointment for relief.

Chapter 7
Medical Conditions Requiring Immediate Help

If you have a common purpose and an environment in which people want to help others succeed, the problems will be fixed quickly.

- Alan Mulally

Some medical conditions require immediate attention. Delaying first aid or waiting for the medical emergency unit may result in a fatality. Although nearly all the medical conditions listed in this chapter require a medical expert's diagnosis, treatment, and even surgery in some cases, a first aider can keep the situation from worsening with some simple yet important procedures.

Heart Attack

A heart attack occurs when there is a sudden decline in the flow of blood to the heart muscle. Usually, is it to blame for clots in the coronary artery which stops the circulation of blood. The biggest risk is the stopping of the heart. A heart attack can vary from person to person and its effects also vary depending on how much damage has been caused. Many people who have had a heart attack never recover fully.

If you suspect someone having a heart attack, confirm it before beginning first aid. Look for these signs and symptoms below:

- Persistent chest pain that spreads from the shoulder up to the jaw and in the left arm.
- Breathlessness
- Collapse
- Discomfort in the stomach like severe indigestion
- The blueness of skin and the lips
- Air hunger (gasping for air)
- Dizziness or fainting
- Feeling impending doom
- A weak or irregular pulse
- Sweating

What to Do?

- First, don't panic.
- Call 911 for help. Let the operator know that you think that the person might be having a heart attack.
- Ask the patient to not panic and remain calm as panicking will only add to the strain on their heart.
- Make the patient lie in a half-sitting position with hands resting on the knees. To add more support to their head and shoulders, put some cushions behind them so that they can sit in a relaxed position. You may also put cushions under their knees.

- Aspirin helps with a heart attack. Help the patient take a full dose of aspirin. Advise them to chew it.

- If the patient is an angina patient, ask if he/she has a pump-action, angina medication or an aerosol spray. If yes, help them take it.

- Let them know that they must rest.

- Monitor their vital signs until help arrives and make sure that their pulse doesn't weaken, or breathing isn't compromised.

Stroke

A stroke is a condition in which the blood supply to the brain stops. Strokes are the third most common cause of death in the US. The effects are long-term and the people who have a stroke mostly live with disabilities resulting from it. People that are at most risk of having a stroke are seniors with high blood pressure. Like a heart attack, during a stroke, a blood clot forms in one of the arteries that stops the flow of blood to the brain. In some rare cases, a rupture in one of the blood vessels can also result in a stroke as it causes a bleed in the brain. In the event of a stroke, the earlier the patient is treated, the lower the chances of life-long damages.

This means that the first aider must be quick to assess the signs and decide on a course of action. One of the best ways to determine if an individual is suffering from a stroke is by using the FAST method. Take a look at what each letter stands for.

- F (Face): This stands for facial weakness. If an individual experiences a facial weakness, meaning they aren't able to smile or open their mouth when told to, they might be having a stroke. The eyes may also become droopy.

- A (Arm): This stands for arm weakness. If someone is having a stroke, they will only be able to raise one of their arms. To confirm your suspicion, ask the person to raise both hands.

- S (Speech): This stands for any complications in being able to speak. When someone has a stroke, they are unable to speak.

- T (Time): This refers to calling the medical emergency services if you have all your suspicions confirmed.

Other signs and symptoms may include:

- Numbness of the face, arms, and legs
- Blurred vision
- Confused state of mind
- Severe headache
- Sudden fall
- Dizziness or unsteadiness

What to Do?

- Call 911 right away. The sooner you get the patient to the hospital, the better. Let the operator know that the patient is having a stroke and needs immediate medical attention. Also, let them know that you used the FAST technique to confirm your suspicions.

- Tell the victim to remain calm. Offer them to lie down and keep their body supported. Remind them often that help is on the way. The goal is to ensure that they keep responding and not lose consciousness.

- Monitor their vital signs, their breathing, and their heart rate. If anything seems out of the ordinary, ask the operator what more you can do.

- Don't let anyone around them offer them something to eat or drink. It will only make it worse if they can't chew or swallow and the food gets stuck in their airways.

Angina

Angina refers to the tightening of the chest. It happens when the arteries that are supposed to supply blood to the heart shrink or narrow, limiting the flow of blood. The less blood they carry, the less blood the heart gets to pump throughout the body. Angina is most often reported in patients that experienced extreme excitement or exertion. Although it isn't as bad as a stroke or a heart attack, it must be taken seriously. Usually, the symptoms of angina go away on their own, but if they continue to persist, you might have mistaken it for angina. The patient could be having a heart attack and thus care must be administered for it right away.

Some of the most common signs and symptoms of someone suffering from angina include:

- Central chest pain that spreads to the jaws and arms
- Pain that goes away with rest
- Feelings of anxiety

- Shortness of breath

- Sudden or extreme fatigue

What to Do?

- Advise the patient to stop whatever they are doing and sit down. Reassure them that this will help with the pain and discomfort.

- Ask the patient if they have angina medication on them. If yes, get it for them. Whether it is a tablet, aerosol spray or pump-action, administer it for them if they are unable to do so themselves.

- Wait for 5 minutes for the medication to work. Meanwhile continue talking to them, reminding them that it will be alright in a few minutes.

- If after 5 minutes, they still complain of chest pains or shortness of breath, ask them to take another dose.

- If they are sitting, ask them to lie down and let any bystanders move away to allow them some space and air.

- If they still report pain after another 5 minutes, call 911. As stated above, it could be a heart attack and require medical assistance right away.

- If the pain subdues after the second dose of medication, the patient should be able to resume what he/she was doing after a while.

Drowning

Drowning can be life-threatening. It can lead to hypothermia in which the individual loses their body's heat sooner than they should. Drowning in cold water can cause the patient to have a cardiac arrest or suffer from throat spasms and airway blockage.

Drowning incidents are quite common during summers and especially among kids who are learning to swim. Even though they are rescued before something bad happens, the trauma can be scary and unforgettable.

If a person has been rescued from drowning, chances are that they need immediate medical attention. Even when they seem to act fine, if the water entered the lungs, it may begin to irritate them after several hours. If that escalates, swelling of the lungs may also be experienced, called secondary drowning.

What to Do?

- Lie them down on a rug or mat with their head slightly lower than the rest of their body. This should help the water drain out from the mouth and reduce the chances of water inhalation.

- Start with the treatment for hypothermia which involves removing their wet clothes and dressing them into dry ones.

- Once the water has been drained and the patient has changed into dry clothes, cover them in blankets or coats to re-instill some heat into the body.

- If the patient is fully responsive, make them something hot to drink.

- If the patient isn't responsive, start with chest compressions and rescue breathing. Check for any signs of breathing and pulse.

- Call 911 and let the operator know of the situation.

- Continue with chest compressions until help arrives.

Dislocation of Bones

Dislocation of joints can be of two types. Either the whole of the bone is removed from its original position or just one end of it. A dislocation occurs when some strong external forces wrench the bone into an abnormal state. Dislocation is most common in shoulders, knees, and fingers. Sometimes only the ligaments are torn. Other times it is the synovial membrane that takes the hit which keeps the bone locked in a capsule.

Like fractures, dislocation of a joint can have serious consequences. A dislocation or slipping of one of the vertebrae can cause permanent damage to the spinal cord. Similarly, a dislocation in the shoulder or hip muscles can damage the large nerves supporting them. A lot of times, it is difficult to identify whether it is a fracture or dislocation. Since fractures are a more serious and life-threatening concern, dislocation must also be treated as a fracture when the true cause is unknown.

What signs should you look for in case of a dislocation?

- Sickening pain like that in a fracture

- Swelling or bruising of the affected area

- Inability to move
- Deformity in the area
- Bent or shortened area

What to Do?

- The first thing to do is ensure that the casualty keeps the dislocated limb steady. Too much movement can trigger excruciating pain as well as discomfort.

- Don't try to reposition it on your own as you may cause more damage. Instead, allow support to the injured region using a cushion or pillow or using a makeshift sling. This is referred to as immobilization of the dislocated injury.

- If the shoulder has been dislocated, create an arm sling that holds the hand of the dislocated shoulder to the chest. This will secure the limb in place and also prevent the movement of the arm.

- Broken bones or dislocation aren't something you can treat at home. The extent of the injury can only be measured with an MRI and X-ray. Thus, the next step should be to drive the casualty to a hospital to have it checked to see if surgery is required.

- If the person starts to go into shock, keep reassuring them that they will be fine. You must keep them calm as anxiety and panic can lead to an increased heart rate and shortness of breath.

- Check for the circulation of blood from time to time in the sling. It shouldn't be too tight as to stop the circulation. A lack of flow will result in swelling as well as drying of the blood vessels and turn the skin bluish.

Seizures

A seizure or convulsion is an involuntary contraction of multiple muscles in the body simultaneously. A seizure happens when there is some disturbance in the electrical activity of our brains. When someone has a seizure, their body shakes vigorously followed by a loss of consciousness.

The most commonly reported cause of seizures is epilepsy. Epilepsy is a neurological disorder that involves recurrent episodes of disturbances in our senses and is accompanied by convulsions or impairment of consciousness. Other causes of a seizure may include brain-damaging diseases, head injury, shortness of oxygen in the body, glucose deficiency or intake of drugs or poisons.

So, you see, seizures aren't a medical condition themselves but rather an indication or warning of an underlying disease. Regardless of that, if someone is having a seizure, they must be attended to at the earliest opportunity before the individual loses consciousness.

During a seizure, the airways get blocked which can lead to poor blood circulation. If the situation escalates, the patient might have a cardiac arrest or stroke. Contrarily, it should pass on its own in a couple of minutes. Thus, monitoring the patient's vitals until medical assistance arrives is a must. If you notice any of these signs and symptoms in the patient, it is a confirmation of a seizure.

- Loss of consciousness suddenly

- Convulsive movements
- An arched back and rigid body
- Difficulty in breathing
- Lips turning blue or gray
- Saliva dripping from the mouth or blood if the casualty has bitten his/her tongue
- Loss of bowel control
- Loss of bladder control
- No recall of the seizure when it passes away
- The patient might want to go to sleep right away

What to Do?

- Let the patient have some space and ask any bystanders to move away.
- If there are any potentially dangerous items on the floor around them, use your legs to remove them in case the patient collapses.
- Note the time the seizure started so that you may call 911 in case it exceeds 2 to 3 minutes.
- Make the patient lie down and put something under their head and neck for support.
- If they are wearing tight clothing, now would be the time to open a few buttons to allow them to breathe easily.

- Wait for the seizure to pass on its own.

- If the seizure passes, check for normal breathing. Ensure that the airways aren't blocked, and the breathing has returned to normal. Put the patient in the recovery position for a few minutes before asking them to stand up.

- Check for vitals such as pulse rate and their verbal response. Note the time of the seizure so you know how long it lasted.

- If the patient continues to shake, call 911 and ask the operator to send help.

Childbirth

Childbirth is a lengthy but natural process that occurs usually after a woman has completed 38+ weeks of pregnancy. Although an ideal time would be 40 weeks, most women give birth any day after the 38th week. Since it takes some time before the child finally enters the world, there is plenty of time to get to the hospital. However, in some cases, the baby decides to arrive unannounced and quickly. If someone around you goes directly into labor or for some reason can't be taken to a hospital, you might want to prepare for an emergency birth at home. With spontaneous births, there is usually excessive bleeding involved but if the right measures are taken, everything can go smoothly.

Birth has three stages. The first stage is when the baby moves into the position for birth. The second stage is when the baby is born, and the third stage is when the placenta and umbilical cord are delivered. In case a woman goes into labor, there is no need to assist her while delivering as it is going to happen naturally. Your role as a first aider should be to keep the woman in labor calm and relaxed.

What to Do

- Call 911 and let them know that the woman is about to deliver and can't be taken to a hospital.

- Let them know of the stage the birthing is in so that they can help you with what you need to do.

- Note the time of each contraction as it will let you estimate how much time is left before the baby finally arrives.

- As the baby's head starts to pop out of the vagina, lay your hand underneath for support. Since there is a lot of mucus, it can become slippery very quickly.

- As soon as the woman makes the final push and you have a newborn in your hands safe, cover them with a clean blanket or piece of cloth.

- Don't tug or pull the umbilical cord to pull the placenta out. Instead, place the baby gently in between the legs of the mother to ease the last few pushes.

- Don't try to cut the umbilical cord. Keep it intact until a nurse or professional arrives.

- Let the mother know that she did an amazing job and congratulate her on becoming one.

The end... almost!

Reviews are not easy to come by.

As an independent author with a tiny marketing budget, I rely on readers, like you, to leave a short review on Amazon.

Even if it's just a sentence or two!

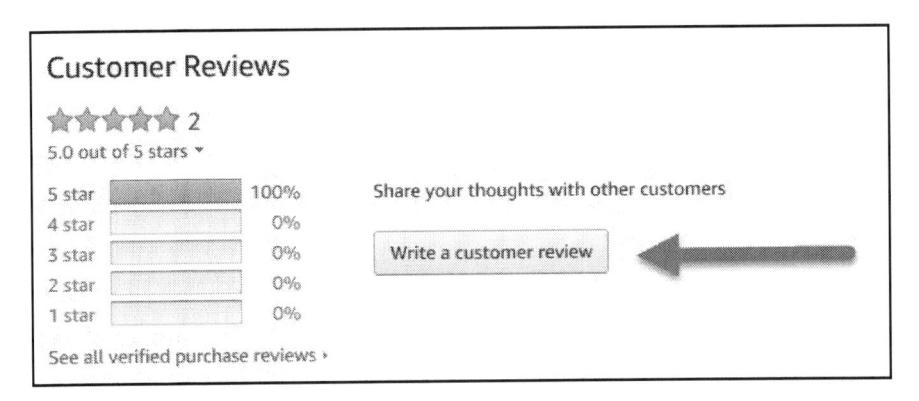

```
Customer Reviews
★★★★★ 2
5.0 out of 5 stars ▼
5 star  ████████ 100%    Share your thoughts with other customers
4 star            0%
3 star            0%     [ Write a customer review ]  ⬅
2 star            0%
1 star            0%
See all verified purchase reviews ›
```

So if you enjoyed the book, please...

\>> Click here to leave a brief review on Amazon.

https://www.amazon.com/review/create-review?asin=B084DHDQWN

I am very appreciative for your review as it truly makes a difference.

Thank you from the bottom of my heart for purchasing this book and reading it to the end.

Final Thoughts

It is necessary to help others, not only in our prayers but in our daily lives. If we find we cannot help others, the least we can do is to desist from harming them.

-Dalai Lama

Accidents happen all the time. They aren't planned or anticipated. There is always a 1% chance that something might not be right. So, are you prepared to deal with that 1% when things get out of hand and someone has an injury?

Rushing an injured person to the hospital might seem like the best option. But it isn't ideal in all cases especially ones where the injured person has a broken bone or can't be moved. The time you waste driving can cost a life. Therefore, it is best to let help come to you rather than you making a run for them in those cases. Meanwhile, you should start administering first aid on your own. But be sure to let 911 know about the emergency.

Administering first aid isn't difficult. The techniques you have learned in this guide will help you tackle some of the most common medical emergencies in your home, workplace and outdoors. You must always be prepared mentally and emotionally to take charge as it can mean saving someone's life.

Don't hesitate in offering help or waiting for someone else to step forward. There are times when the difference between life and death is merely a few minutes.

With an increase in road accidents, climate-related calamities, and in-home injuries, everyone should be aware of some basic techniques to help the people around them. If you follow all the techniques discussed in this book to a tee, there is no need to worry about the outcome of the situation. At least you will know in your heart that you tried your best and did everything you could.

DOWNLOAD YOUR FREE GIFT BELOW:

These 14 New Habits Will Double Your Income, from Today

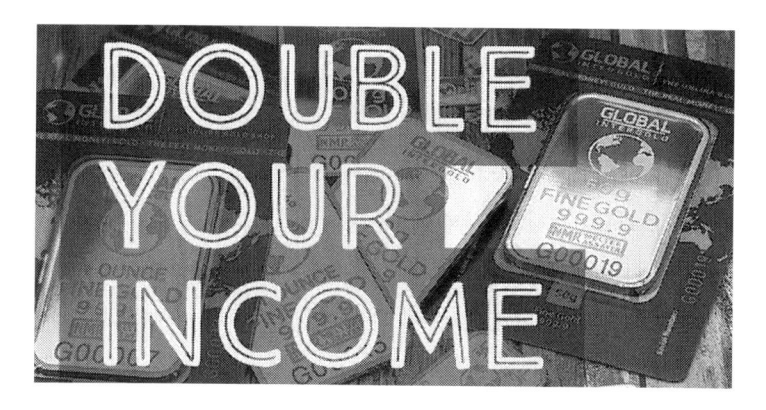

An Easy Cheat Sheet to Adopting 14 Powerful Success Habits:

Stop Procrastinating and Start Earning with Intent Now!

Are Your Bad Habits Keeping You from the Life You Want?

Mine definitely were, but then I dedicated myself to new habits

– and everything changed!

Most people get stuck in same old routines. We eat the same breakfast, we talk to the same people. Human beings are creatures of habit, and it locks us into negative cycles we don't even know are there. Like me, you've had enough of the same-old, same-old. It's time for change!

This guide gives you the 14 most high impact habits that helped me double my income nearly instantly, when I set out on this journey. I will help you change, and I'll make it stick!

This FREE Cheat Sheet contains:

- Daily success habits that the most successful people in the world live by

- Common, but little-known habits that will surprise you

- Details on what Stephen Covey, Oprah Winfrey, Elon Musk, Bill Gates and Albert Einstein did that you aren't doing to maximize your earning potential

- Tips on how to overcome habit fatigue

- The reality of adopting difficult, challenging habits and the rewards that result

Scroll below and click the link to claim your cheat sheet!

It's tough to admit that you're doing it wrong. I went through it, and it sucks. After that I was free to change however necessary, to meet my goals. I want you to know that change is waiting for you. This guide is so easy to follow, and if you put it to work in your life – you will double your income.

Adopt these habits, and change your life.

CLICK HERE!!

Check out our Other *AMAZING* Titles:

Book 1: <u>Dealing With Dementia and Alzheimer's:</u>

<u>Your Guide to Coping With and Caring for a Loved One</u>

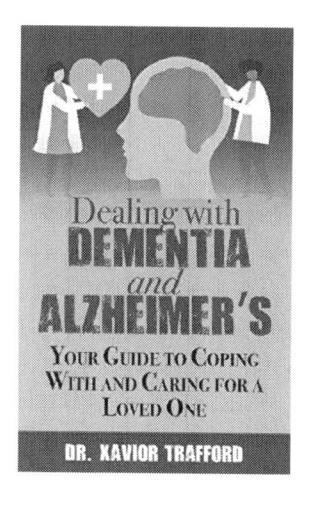

Planning and Logistics

Planning and preparation of legal documents needs to begin as soon as you've received a diagnosis. It will seem almost cold-hearted to do all of this, but you need to sit down with your loved one and explain everything that is going to happen and also explain what the doctor has just said. It helps to have the doctor or a trusted third-party advisor, like a nurse, present when you're having this conversation.

In terms of legalities, the amount of work you'll need to do depends on the state of your loved one. Often this is simply a case of taking care of a few standard documents and you're good to go. The sections in this chapter will address all the broad categories of things that need to be taken care of.

Legal Matters

This category contains the largest number of things you will have to take or including financial assets. It is very important that you prepare all legal documents as soon as possible. The reason for this is due to the fact that legal professionals rely on a concept called "capacity" when preparing documents. Capacity is a person's ability to understand the nature of the document they're signing (Sauer, 2018).

Power of Attorneys

You will find that a lot of lawyers will refuse to prepare legal documents for people who have received a diagnosis of dementia or AD. This is especially the case with AD. While this seems a bit harsh, there are lawyers who will prepare documents for people in the early stages of the disease provided they can demonstrate capacity.

Patients in the middle or late stages of AD lose the ability to do so, which is why you should organize everything as quickly as possible. The following documents need to be prepared, at a minimum:

1. Durable power of attorney

2. Healthcare power of attorney

3. Living will or trusts

4. Financial statement of accounts

5. Will

All of these documents need to be prepared with the consent and in the presence of the person suffering from AD. It helps to involve them in the process and empowers them as well since it removes the patient from the feeling of helplessness they will experience. The durable power of attorney enables a person to make decisions on behalf of the patient, including all financial ones.

The healthcare power of attorney is not something to be taken lightly. This empowers a person to act on behalf of the patient if they are incapacitated when it comes to deciding medication and end of life matters. If you're the sole person who will be in charge of both documents, then you need to have an in-depth discussion with your loved one about what sort of facilities they will want, especially when it comes to the end of life care.

Have a deep discussion between yourselves as best as you can and then discuss it briefly in front of your lawyer so that they can see that the patient understands what the document is and the consequences of what is being discussed. In addition to the healthcare power of attorney, you should draft a living will. The living will document grants medical professionals permission to remove a person of life support equipment in case of incapacitation so that the patient may pass away naturally.

Financial Aspects

A living trust is a financial document that needs to be prepared in conjunction with a will. A person needs to be appointed as the legal guardian and this person needs to meet with a qualified financial advisor to review the financial position of the patient. Collect all bank statements, records, and investment statements, including tax filings, and meet with them.

In case of large assets, it is best to work with an estate planner who can walk you through all the consolidation options available. There will be tax issues to consider so these need to be handled as well. This is also the time for you to map out medical expenses, which I'll talk about in the next section.

In case your budget is tight and finances are an issue, approaching a nearby senior center will help if doing the research yourself seems problematic or risky. Senior centers usually have contacts with lawyers practicing in what is called Elder Law. Elder law deals with all sorts of aspects of senior care planning, including estate planning, disability planning, guardianship, Medicare planning and social security benefits.

Obtaining guardianship for your loved one is a process that involves the courts. Usually, a court psychologist determines whether the person in question is truly incapacitated or not and presents their findings to the court. This is the easy bit. The hard part is convincing the judge that you are a worthy guardian. So, prepare to have your financial statements and plans scrutinized.

The court will want to hear your plans for medical care, such as how you intend to support your loved one and whether you'll need to cut back on the hours at your existing job and or source of income.

Hiring a competent elder law attorney will help immensely with all of this. The most scrutinized portion of the application will have to do with money. If you've borrowed some money from them and have made transactions which don't pass scrutiny or are questionable, expect the process to get a lot harder. It is best to let your attorney know of all these things well in advance.

Emergency Guardianship

Guardianship is not an urgent process unless your loved one is in the final stages of AD or dementia and there have been no measures placed at this time. The other scenario which requires you to consider emergency guardianship is when your loved one is being taken advantage of by a scam artist.

Scammers regularly target the elderly who do not have the capacity to make their own decisions and will financially exploit them. This will be a contentious hearing because your loved one will likely rebel against your plans, but you need to see it through nonetheless.

Hiring an Attorney

Before hiring an attorney, gather all of you and your loved one's legal documents and make sure they're in order. The best method of finding a reasonable attorney is through a referral. Elder law attorneys also work at large law firms and there are a lot of positives in choosing a large firm over an independent lawyer. Firstly, there are likely to be a number of financial issues that you'll need help with and a large law firm likely has all of the experts under a single roof.

However, this doesn't mean the solitary attorney cannot get the job done. Check with them to see what sorts of connections they have when you meet with them for a consultation. A good place to find elder law attorneys is to head over to the National Academy of Elder Law Attorneys (NAELA) ("5 Tips for Choosing a Good Elder Law Attorney," 2018). Their website even helps you find attorneys close to you.

Before meeting the attorney, send them a summary of what you're looking for and summarize the current legal position. Once you do this, most attorneys will be willing to meet with you for free. Meet multiple attorneys and check their references. Compare their advice and evaluate the person you feel most comfortable working with.

Experience is the key here and you may probably know that by now. Experience also means your lawyer will have connections in the area which can come in handy when you need some service that falls outside their legal circle of competence. No single lawyer can specialize in everything so check to see how good your attorney's network is as mentioned previously.

Lastly, head onto the state bar association's website to see if the person is licensed to practice and if they're registered. This should be a formality, but it never hurts to check. If you find that you cannot afford an attorney, then you do have some options available to you.

The first is to contact the LegalAid, which is a nonprofit organization with offices across the United States. Beware that there are income qualifications (as in you need to be below a certain limit) and you need to be truly in need in order to qualify ("5 Tips for Choosing a Good Elder Law Attorney," 2018). Check for any community legal aid programs in your area as these often offer free services as part of pro bono work from larger law firms. Lawhelp.org is a website you can use to find pro bono programs in your area as well.

Medical Matters

Your doctor is going to decide what sort of treatment plan will be appropriate. This decision will be based on the stage of dementia your loved one is in, their age and medical history, and your preferences. Generally, if your doctor decides to prescribe drugs it will likely be one of the following:

6. Aricept - This is the only drug that has been FDA approved for every stage of AD (Legg, 2019).

7. Razadyne - This works for mild to medium stages of dementia.

8. Exlon - Similar to Razadyne, this can even be ingested via a skin patch.

9. Memantine - This drug is prescribed for moderate to severe AD. It inhibits the production of a chemical that is produced as a result of the disease. It is usually prescribed in conjunction with one of the other drugs mentioned.

10. Namzaric - This is for those patients who have severe symptoms and for whom previous medication has not worked.

Despite the impressive-sounding list of names, you must understand that all of these only slow down the symptoms and not the disease itself. There is no cure for AD and you and your loved one need to consider the side effects of ingesting all of these drugs. Common side effects include dizziness, nausea, and diarrhea. Make sure your doctor explains everything to you in detail and make an informed choice. If your loved one is not in a position to express their wishes, then this is a tough choice. In such cases, it's best to go with what the doctor suggests.

Your doctor might also suggest taking part in clinical trials that go a long way in developing a cure for the disease. It is helpful to take part in these, but thus far, there have been no significant advancements in determining a treatment for AD.

Costs

Aside from all of those prescriptions, you need to take into account how much care your loved one is going to cost you. In the United States, care for a person with AD is estimated to be $329,360 over the lifetime of that patient ("Know What to Expect", 2019). It is also estimated that 70% of this cost is borne out of pocket by the family. These are not insignificant sums when you consider that the average AD patient lives for an average of five to eight years after their initial diagnosis.

The majority of this cost goes towards patient care as opposed to drugs, which is why a lot of it isn't covered. This is why it's essential to sit down with your loved one and talk things out while they're still capable. The last thing they want is to leave you with debt. No matter what your sense of duty tells you to do, it's important to discuss things out in detail.

During these conversations, it is important to get a grasp of what their general idea is about how they want things to go. While their general directives might not cover every possible scenario, it helps doctors immensely if you were able to express your loved one's wishes with regard to a situation. So, get to know their philosophy and what they would want to be done in a particular situation.

Another important topic of discussion is to talk about if they wish to live with their family. As their condition deteriorates, you will have to consider placing them in an assisted living facility and this has both emotional and financial ramifications. This will be a tough conversation, but you need to consider the financial aspect as well of any decision that emanates from this.

In addition to this, if your loved one has a considerable financial net worth, you should determine what percentage of this needs to be directed toward their healthcare and how much should be left as part of their will. Your loved one should also leave behind a clear plan as to what must happen to their assets and liabilities as applicable. The will or trust will usually cover this ground.

You should also consider convincing them to sign up for long term care (LTC) insurance. Traditional LTC plans work like a regular insurance plan and are paid off when you need assistance with daily tasks. However, thanks to faulty underwriting practices, the industry was forced to reassess limits and now offers what is called a hybrid LTC. This type of LTC results in a payout if your loved one doesn't end up needing to use the care benefits. Thus, it works like a mini life insurance policy, which can be beneficial to cover any emergency costs.

Do note that the premiums of traditional LTCs are cheaper than the hybrid ones for obvious reasons. However, given their lump sum payout potential at the end, it is an option worth considering.

Safety and Your Home

After the initial diagnosis, people normally choose to have their loved ones move in with them. This poses a unique challenge since you now need to AD proof your home. Even if your loved one suffers from another form of dementia, there are significant risks you need to mitigate in order to make the environment as safe and comfortable as possible for them.

A lot of seniors who suffer from dementia begin to neglect taking care of themselves thanks to safety hazards posing a challenge. So, work your way through the checklist below and ensure this doesn't happen.

Prep Hotspots

There are certain areas in your home which are going to be potentially hazardous for your loved one. These are garages, workrooms, basements, or areas where tools and chemicals are stored. Store cleaning supplies under lock and key, and make sure none of these places are easily accessible. Basements especially pose a double threat thanks to stairs and dim lighting.

You should ensure these areas are well lit but leaving the lights on at all times is not practical. Hence, simply ensure that things are locked securely and that none of your family members leaves doors open by mistake.

Kitchens

The kitchen is another literal hot zone. Install safety valves to ensure that they cannot switch the gas on by mistake or, as is more common, forget to turn the gas off which will lead to a massive fire hazard. The best thing to do is to remove all knobs from your stove and when purchasing new appliances, consider getting ones that have an auto shut off feature.

In addition to this, remove any decorations or falling hazards you might be using for visual purposes. Things like decorative fruits and so on are an example of this.

Know Your Numbers

Keep a list of emergency numbers taped to your refrigerator at all times. Save it into your phone. Write it onto a post-it and keep it in an accessible place where your loved one can see it clearly. Remember to include your own number in there or create a separate note with just your number on it so that they can reach you immediately. While in the later stages it is a long shot that they'll remember where these notes are, consider hanging a sketchpad and writing your number on it prominently so that they can see it easily.

Check Your Safety Devices

Have professionals evaluate your home's smoke detectors, fire alarms, extinguishers and so on. Consider installing them if you don't have them already. A lot of homes don't have carbon monoxide detectors installed, for example. Check with your home security provider if there's any additional precautionary programs they can offer you if you can afford it.

Install Locks Wisely

Place locks well out of reach in different places. So, install them either high or low on the door and do not have any locks on the inside since they're likely to lock themselves in. This is especially the case with bathrooms, so figure out how they can have their privacy but also be safe at the same time.

Keep an extra set of keys for everything in a place where they can be accessed easily by you. Make sure the doors that lead to the outside your home are secured and that your loved one cannot open them and wander off by mistake.

Light it Up

Ensure the walkways and stairs in your home are well lit and that all the bulbs work. Add more lamps if need be, especially if your loved one suffers from poor eyesight. A good way of inducing visual cognition without flooding everything in light is to simply paint the walls a different color. This is especially true for bathrooms which tend to be monotone.

Painting the walls and the floor a different color, something bright preferably, will help your loved one differentiate between them and will create a nice contrast as well.

Remove Any Weapons

Disable the triggers on all weapons inside your home since this is a genuine hazard. If your loved one forgets who you are, as is likely, unfortunately, they might mistake you for an intruder and attack you. Place all sharp objects such as knives or tools in a locked drawer and keep the keys well out of their reach.

Store Medication

Place all medication and other medical information or devices in a securely locked drawer. Use a pillbox and monitor the dosage. You will likely need to give them their medication personally since they're likely to forget to take it or mix up their dosage. So, you will need to figure out how you're going to make this work if it conflicts with your regular schedule.

Tripping Hazards

Remove all clutter from your home which might pose a tripping hazard. The living room is usually the place for these so as tasteful your new decor might look, make it safe. Things like floor lamps or glass vases need to be placed somewhere else. Also, watch out for sharp-edged tables or furniture which they might absentmindedly bump into.

Bathrooms are a major area of tripping hazards, so purchase grip mats and even buy them footwear that maximizes grip within your home. When using the kitchen, pay special attention to where you place hot food since they might not be able to tell when something is hot. In addition to grip mats, place grab bars in showers or tubs. You might need to consider reinstalling some of your bathroom fixtures or modifying them in a particular location.

It might be tempting to go to an extreme and make your home too restrictive. Put your modifications in place and check to see how well they cope with it. You don't want to turn your home into jail, so seek to strike the right balance. Above all else, remember that they need to be comfortable as well as safe.

Book 2: Intermittent Fasting for Women

The Complete Guide to Healthy Eating for Weight Loss and Body Cleansing

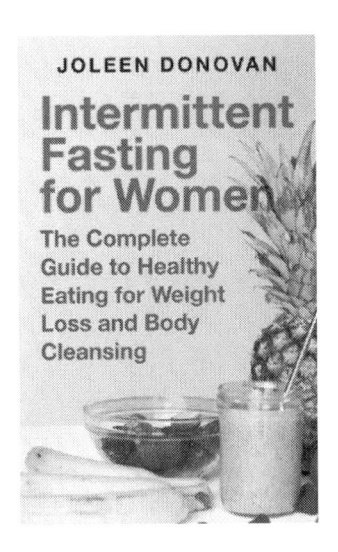

Science Behind Intermittent Fasting

While every diet and fitness addition into your life comes with upsides and downsides, intermittent fasting has more pros than cons. If you approach intermittent fasting with an open mind, you'll find that it can help you reach your weight loss goals. In the next part more will be shared about the science behind intermittent fasting and what you can do about your hunger while fasting.

There is plenty of information and research that backs up intermittent fasting. As fasting is not a new thing, extensive research can be found on this topic. Intermittent fasting may soon become a fad, but thankfully it is a fad that is based on science. While much of the research on fasting has been done on animals, the science is still promising.

Fasting is not a new phenomenon. Fasting has been shown in the past to help the body to reset and clear the mind. Interestingly, science goes far beyond that. While there are several different theories as to why intermittent fasting works, one fascinating theory that has been well-researched is that intermittent fasting puts your body's cells under mild stress. When these cells are stressed, they keep adapting and can fight off disease better. Stress is something that often carries a negative connotation.

On the contrary, stress is not inherently a bad thing. When you put your body under stress, positive results can occur. Think of when you exercise hard. You are exhausted and tired, but once your muscles recover, they are stronger. Research has shown that your body's cells respond to intermittent fasting very similar to exercise.

The reason you will lose weight while intermittent fasting can be attributed to a few different causes. For one, it will be much easier to eat fewer calories in the limited eating window. If you are eating on alternate days, during a window period, or skipping certain meals, you will tend to be consuming fewer calories than when you were eating multiple meals throughout the day. Another reason you may lose weight while fasting is because when you stop eating for an extended period, your body goes into its adipose tissue fat cells for energy. Ketones are released into the bloodstream that carries fat, and you end up losing your body fat through your urine. Research also shows that short-term fasting increases your metabolism speed. Your metabolism is what digests your food. When it works faster, it burns more calories, leading to more weight loss. While many other diets may limit your calorie intake, intermittent fasting does both things. You increase the calories you expend (by boosting your metabolism), and you also decrease the calories you eat. This creates a large calorie deficit. If you exercise on top of intermittent fasting, your calorie deficit becomes larger, and you will lose even more weight.

Intermittent fasting did not become a craze just because of weight loss. Intermittent fasting is popular amongst many already fit individuals because of the other benefits it comes with. One of these benefits is reducing the chance of insulin resistance. Type two diabetes is on the rise. Research says that intermittent fasting leads to a drop in blood sugar levels. Fasting, insulin was seen to drop as much as 20-30% and fasting blood sugar dropped by 3-6%. When you have lower insulin and blood sugar levels, you are at a lower risk for developing insulin resistance, which leads to type two diabetes.

If you are looking for anti-aging benefits, intermittent fasting may be the diet for you, too. Our bodies go through a process called oxidative stress. Oxidative stress leads to aging and many of the chronic diseases that we see on the rise today. Harmful free radicals react with our body's proteins and DNA and damage them which leads to these diseases and aging. However, studies have shown that intermittent fasting increases our body's ability to attack these harmful free radicals. This can help us to combat the effects of aging.

Fasting is also good for the heart. It's no surprise that cardiovascular disease is currently the number one killer in many countries. Intermittent fasting can help stabilize the brain's hormones and brings about better heart health. Fasting can reduce the risk of heart problems with risk factors such as LDL cholesterol, blood triglycerides, blood sugar levels, and inflammation levels lowered. If you have high cholesterol or are on medication for cholesterol and high blood pressure, intermittent fasting could lead to you dropping this medication.

While not proven in humans yet, intermittent fasting has shown impressive benefits in preventing cancer in animal studies. When these animals underwent intermittent fasting, they survived longer and had a reduction in symptoms from their tumors. Cancer is a disease that is not entirely understood and any research showing that this diet can help prevent it should be taken seriously. There was also a study that looked at humans going through chemotherapy. They found that the individuals who followed an intermittent fasting diet had fewer side effects from the chemotherapy. More research will need to be studied to understand fasting's relationship with cancer, but so far it seems to be very positive.

There have many good effects shown throughout research on intermittent fasting but how does it work? How does intermittent fasting cause all these great benefits?

Just as calories from vegetables are better than calories from chocolate cake, the timing of meal consumption can affect how a human body stores it most efficiently. Usually, when we eat something, our metabolism spends hours burning through this food and digesting it. As the stomach digests this food, it will either use the energy or store the energy as fat. Hence, for someone constantly eating throughout the day, the body is going to use the nearest energy source. It is going to burn the calories of what was just eaten instead of the stored energy from body fat. It doesn't need body fat because it is constantly getting a new stream of energy from the food that is being consumed 3 or more times a day. With intermittent fasting, the body is not provided with consistent food at every few hour intervals. Hence, with the body realizing it is not receiving any food, it starts to burn the calories from stored energy, or fat cells. These fat cells become the only energy source available and therefore are being burned from the body.

This can also happen with one workout while practicing intermittent fasting. During the process of fasting and post-workout, the body does not have enough glucose and glycogen to draw from due to a meal skipped. So instead of burning through carbohydrates, where glucose and glycogen often come from, it is forced to look inward for energy. The easiest energy available is the fat stored in adipose tissue. This helps one to lose weight and become leaner. However, intermittent fasting does not stop there. It also aims to make one more sensitive to insulin. When we eat, our body produces insulin. Many individuals are becoming resistant to insulin because of frequent and short eating intervals on top of the high glycemic index food consumed. The more one eats the more insulin that needs to be produced. While insulin is not inherently bad, if the person is not sensitive enough to insulin, he or she will never feel full and keep eating. Fasting changes how we produce and react to insulin. Due to the lesser amount of food consumed, our body is going to release less insulin. The more insulin sensitive one is, the better the body can store the calories consumed. When one breaks fast and starts eating, the body will either use up that energy immediately, store little of it, or it will be converted to glycogen and stored in muscles for use later. Insulin is what is causing many people to gain weight. This insulin resistance is leading to overweight people and many different diseases. With intermittent fasting reducing insulin fluctuations and production, it creates a bunch of other great benefits.

Book 3: <u>Bodyweight Training Focusing Your Mind to Transform Your Body</u>

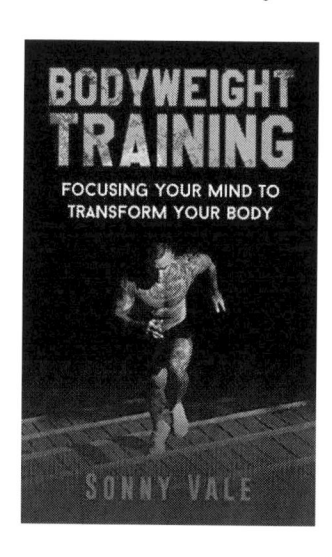

Bodyweight Training; Getting Started

Now that you are convinced about the reasons why you should try bodyweight training, where should you start? Do you know how the exercises differ? Should you begin with full body workouts? Well, there is no doubt that one can easily get confused when kicking off their training program. This happens because various routines need to be performed. It is also easy to get stuck along the way as one could be bored with the routines that they have been performing. This is the main reason why you should have a program. A program helps you in knowing what you should train and at what time. This program guides you in ensuring that you balance your workouts for optimum results. But before you design a training program, you first have to understand

Full Body

The exercises discussed here are classified as full body exercises. This implies that they aid in developing your entire body.

Inchworm

Begin this exercise with your legs straight. Next, lower your torso as you try to get your fingertips to hit the ground. While in this position, try to walk your hands forward as though you want to perform push-ups. Don't perform any push-ups. However, move back to the initial position that you were in at the beginning of the exercise. Your last position should be where your fingertips meet your feet again. Repeat the exercise for about 4 to 6 reps.

Tuck Jump

Just as the name suggests, this exercise requires that you jump with your legs tucked in. So, begin with a jumping position. Jump and try to tuck in your legs so that your arms reach them. Your landing position should be with your knees slightly bent. Repeat the exercise for 3-6 reps while ensuring that the jumping and landing positions are maintained.

Mountain Climber

Picture a scenario where an individual is climbing a steep mountain. This exercise is done in the same manner. Your initial position should be similar to the push-ups position. Next, bring your right foot towards your armpits. This should be done while ensuring that your left leg is straightened. While doing this, it is also important to work on your stomach muscles; they should be kept tight. Switch the legs and perform the same exercise all over again.

Stair Climb

The stairs in your home or around your neighborhood could be transformed into a cardio machine. Walk up and down without stopping. This could be done while holding something heavy. The objects that you hold on both hands should be of equal weight to give you balance. Training experts also recommend that stair climb exercises could be combined with bicep curls. This guarantees that the entire body is trained.

Prone Walk

Begin this exercise with your hands and feet on the ground. Your stomach muscles should be kept tight while performing this exercise. With your hands and feet on the ground, move your hands forward. Your toes should not move. Next, move back to your starting position and repeat the exercise. Remember, your starting position should be as though you want to perform push-ups.

Burpees

Burpees is regarded as one among the best full body workout exercises. Begin with a squatting position. Your hands should touch the floor in this position. Next, try to obtain a push-up position by kicking your feet backward. After that, perform a single push-up and return to your low squat position again. Jump up as high as possible and land on a low squat position again. Three sets should be enough if you are a beginner. For expert athletes, performing up to 6 reps will get your heart pumping fast.

Legs

The exercises discussed in this section will help you train your legs while making sure you gain strength and cut down on some calories.

Wall Sit

The exercise is as simple as it sounds. Assume you are sitting on a chair while doing this exercise. Have your back mounted on the wall and slide down to obtain a sitting position. Your final position should be where the thighs are parallel to the floor. Each set should last for 60 seconds. If you wish to add some fire into this exercise, perform some bicep curls.

Lunge

Begin this exercise with your feet apart and your hands on the hips. Next, take a huge step forward with your left leg without moving the right leg. Bring the right leg to the floor by lowering it. Your left leg should still be in the initial position that you took. At this position, the left leg should be in front whereas the right leg should be close to the floor. Return to a standing position and perform the same routine with your right leg taking a step. After doing the same routine with both legs, this is counted as one rep. Strive to hit 10 reps for optimum results.

Lunge Jump

Lunge jump is similar to the lunge exercise described in the above section. Begin with your feet together and move your right foot ahead.

Aim for a lunge position and jump up. Switch your legs before touching the ground so that you land with your left leg ahead. With this exercise, it would be as though you are performing a lunge exercise but in the air.

Squat

The squat is perhaps the master of all exercises when it comes to leg training. Stand with your feet apart. Slowly, crouch to a position where your feet are parallel to the floor. While doing this, confirm that you do not lift your heels. Next, aim to get to a standing position again. Do this ten times and rest. Repeat the exercise.

Calf Raises

This is a simple exercise that gets your feet toned. While in a standing position, rise to the point where your toes hold your body. Your knees should be kept straight and that your heels should be off the floor. Maintain the position briefly before slowly returning to your initial position. Repeat the process.

Back and Chest

Push-up

Without question, this is one of the best classic exercises to start with. Most people would argue that they know how to perform this exercise, but it is still worth the mention. So, begin with both your hands on the floor. Your stomach should be off the ground and core tightened. Next, bend your elbows to get your chest to the floor. Return to the initial position and repeat the process. For a beginner, it is recommended that they should try 7-9 reps.

Donkey Kick

Exercising is all about bringing your wild side into your training program. This is the best way in which you will have fun training. For this exercise, take a push-ups position. This time around, your legs should be together. While maintaining this position, kick both legs behind. Your knees should be slightly bent while doing this. To prevent any injuries, try your best to land gently.

Dolphin Push-up

Do you know how to take a dolphin pose? Well, one thing with exercises is that different trainers would have varying names for the exercises that they perform. Nevertheless, the most important thing is how you perform them. In this case, take a push-up position. Your elbows should hold you off from the ground. While in this position, move your body to the front and up. Your head should rise above your shoulders. Return to your starting position and repeat the process.

Shoulders and Arms

Dips

These exercises will help in toning your triceps. It is for this reason that they are sometimes referred to as triceps dips. Find a bench to sit on and have something that will hold your feet above the ground. The point is to have the entire body off the ground. While holding the bench that you are sitting on, lower your body with your arms. Reach a point where the arms are bent 90 degrees parallel to the floor. Return to the initial position and repeat the exercise for the best results.

Arm Circles

Perhaps this is an exercise that you performed during your P.E. class. Well, it is as simple as it sounds. Simply stand up with your arms fully opened. Try to make clockwise circles with the body in an upright position. Reverse the movement to make sure that both left and right arms are worked on.

From the look of things, these exercises are simple. They are the common exercises that you might have performed before. However, one important thing to remember is that the right form or movement should always be adhered to. Failure to do this could lead to unexpected injuries. Also, it is worth noting that the exercises should not be overlooked regardless of how simple they might be. Focus on training with a goal in mind. You want to keep fit and gain strength. Therefore, do not assume anything.

References

10 Basic First Aid Training Tips & Procedures for Any Emergency. (n.d.). Retrieved from https://unchartedsupplyco.com/blogs/news/basic-first-aid.

Baker, S. (2018, October 11). First-Aid Kits in the Office: What You Need and How to Manage It. Retrieved from https://thebenefitsguide.com/first-aid-kits-office-need-manage/.

Bon, C. A. (18 Sep 2018). Cardiopulmonary resuscitation (CPR). Retrieved October 17, 2019 from https://emedicine.medscape.com/article/1344081-overview

Boseley, S. (2012, September 17). Lack of first-aid skills kills as many as cancer, claims advert. Retrieved October 17, 2019, from https://www.theguardian.com/society/2012/sep/17/first-aid-deaths-tv-campaign

Brouhard, R. (2019, October 6). Are You Ready to Do CPR? Retrieved from https://www.verywellhealth.com/how-to-do-cpr-1298446.

Brouhard, R. (2019, September 29). Learn the Basic First Aid Procedures You Should Know. Retrieved from https://www.verywellhealth.com/basic-first-aid-procedures-1298578.

First Aid Techniques - St John Ambulance. (n.d.). Retrieved from http://www.sja.org.uk/sja/first-aid-advice/first-aid-techniques.aspx.

Hepler, L. (2018, August 3). How to Perform CPR: Hands-Only and Mouth-to-Mouth. Retrieved from https://www.healthline.com/health/first-aid/cpr#steps-for-hands--only-cpr.

How to Recognize Emergencies. (n.d.). Retrieved from https://firstaidcourse101.blogspot.com/2010/08/how-to-recognize-emergencies.html.

Infectious Diseases and Hygiene Procedures. (n.d.). Retrieved from http://www.gsa.ac.uk/media/1026151/First-Aid-Infectious-Diseases-and-Hygiene-Procedures.pdf.

Lee, D. (2019, September 6). How to Bandage a Wound During First Aid. Retrieved from https://www.wikihow.com/Bandage-a-Wound-During-First-Aid.

Projects, C. to W. (2019, September 9). First Aid/Protective Precautions. Retrieved from https://en.wikibooks.org/wiki/First_Aid/Protective_Precautions.

Sweet, D. (2019, June 26). Checklist for a Camping First Aid Kit. Retrieved from https://www.tripsavvy.com/first-aid-checklist-for-camping-498450.

Virtual College. (2019, July 12). First Aid: Types of Bandages. Retrieved from https://www.virtual-college.co.uk/news/health-and-safety/2017/10/first-aid-types-of-bandages.

Workplace First Aid Kit Contents and Supplies Checklist - First Aid - St John Ambulance. (n.d.). Retrieved from http://www.sja.org.uk/sja/first-aid-advice/first-aid-techniques/workplace-first-aid-kit.aspx.

Printed in Great Britain
by Amazon